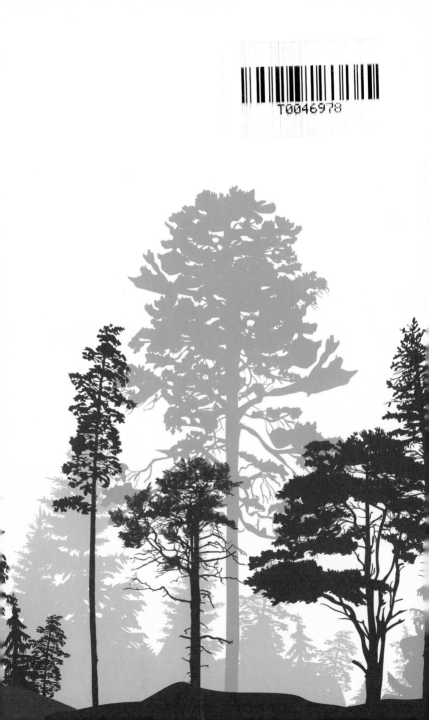

FOREST
BATHING

Note: Shinrin-yoku is considered to be preventive medicine. We emphasize "preventive" because it should never replace official medical advice in case of illness. If you are being treated for an illness, always check with your physician or medical specialist.

To my friend Carlos, with whom I share the dream
of living in a cabin in the mountains of Japan.

—Héctor García

To all the people who fight to save our extraordinary planet,
our only home in the cosmic darkness.

—Francesc Miralles

FOREST BATHING

The Rejuvenating Practice of Shinrin Yoku

Héctor García
and Francesc Miralles

translated from Spanish by Kymm Coveney

TUTTLE Publishing

Tokyo | Rutland, Vermont | Singapore

THE TUTTLE STORY
"Books to Span the East and West"

Our core mission at Tuttle Publishing is to create books which bring people together one page at a time. Tuttle was founded in 1832 in the small New England town of Rutland, Vermont (USA). Our fundamental values remain as strong today as they were then—to publish best-in-class books informing the English-speaking world about the countries and peoples of Asia. The world has become a smaller place today and Asia's economic, cultural and political influence has expanded, yet the need for meaningful dialogue and information about this diverse region has never been greater. Since 1948, Tuttle has been a leader in publishing books on the cultures, arts, cuisines, languages and literatures of Asia. Our authors and photographers have won numerous awards and Tuttle has published thousands of books on subjects ranging from martial arts to paper crafts. We welcome you to explore the wealth of information available on Asia at www.tuttlepublishing.com.

Published by Tuttle Publishing, an imprint of Periplus Editions (HK) Ltd.

www.tuttlepublishing.com

Copyright © 2020 by Héctor García and Francesc Miralles

Originally published in Spanish as *Shinrin Yoku: El Arte Japonés De Sumergirte En La* by Editorial Planeta, Barcelona 2019
Translation rights arranged by Sandra Bruna Agencia Literaria, SL.
All rights reserved.

Translation copyright © 2020 by Periplus Editions (HK) Ltd.

ISBN: 978-4-8053-1600-9

Library of Congress publication data is in progress.

Distributed by

North America, Latin America & Europe
Tuttle Publishing
364 Innovation Drive, North Clarendon,
VT 05759-9436, USA
Tel: 1 (802) 773 8930; Fax: 1 (802) 773 6993
info@tuttlepublishing.com
www.tuttlepublishing.com

Japan
Tuttle Publishing
Yaekari Bldg., 3rd Floor
5-4-12 Osaki, Shinagawa-ku
Tokyo 141 0032
Tel: (81) 3 5437 0171; Fax: (81) 3 5437 0755
sales@tuttle.co.jp
www.tuttle.co.jp

Asia Pacific
Berkeley Books Pte Ltd
3 Kallang Sector #04-01/02
Singapore 349278
Tel: (65) 6280 1330; Fax: (65) 6280 6290
inquiries@periplus.com.sg
www.tuttlepublishing.com

23 22 21 20   6 5 4 3 2 1
Printed in Malaysia   2002VP

TUTTLE PUBLISHING® is a registered trademark of Tuttle Publishing, a division of Periplus Editions (HK) Ltd.

Contents

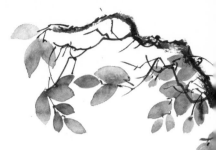

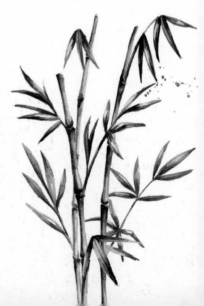

> *"There is nothing you can see that it is not a flower;*
> *there is nothing you can think that it is not the moon."*
> —Matsuo Basho

A Green Twig in Your Heart

The seed for this book was planted in the forests of Hakone, a small city in Kanagawa Prefecture. After our book *Ikigai* divulged the secrets of Japanese centenaries to readers in many parts of the world, we decided to take a trip with some friends and get as far away from Japanese cities as possible, with a mind to exploring the region's wilderness and lakes. We shared a house high in a leafy forest with a well-known psychologist, a biologist, and a philosopher.

The next morning—having slept on the floor, as is still the custom in traditional Japanese homes—we discovered that what the owner of the property had promised us was true. From the veranda, Mount Fuji was clearly visible in all its splendor. We couldn't take our eyes off that mythical, snow-capped summit, so after breakfast we made green tea and took out the musical instruments we'd brought along to do some singing and songwriting on our trip.

We makeshift minstrels had only a small Casio keyboard, a guitalele (half guitar and half ukulele) and our own voices. Inspired by the views of Lake Hakone and by the thick carpeting of trees that surrounded the sacred mountain, we began to lightheartedly improvise a simple song:

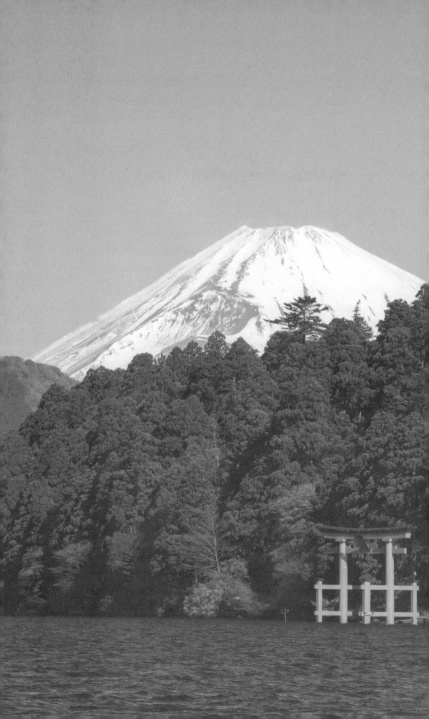

Good morning Fuji,
Green mountains,
Blue sky.
Hello Mount Fuji,
Sometimes shy,
Hiding behind clouds.
Hello Fuji,
White snow,
It is your hat.[1]

Buoyed by the tea and that silly song, we left to take a walk through the majestic forests that led all the way down to the lake. All five of us had accumulated a year's worth of stress caused by our relentless lives in the city where our calendars were chock full of commitments, and obligations seemed to stampede over us in an already overcrowded, polluted environment. This heavy load disappeared as if by magic as soon as we entered the forest. We'd decided to disconnect our cell phones, and as we stepped into the thick woods, a deeply longed-for serenity took hold of us.

We walked slowly, watching the play of sunlight on the branches, mindful of the subtle symphony of nature's sounds and smells. An obstinate cicada practiced its solo to the accompaniment of birdsong and the delicate wind section of a smooth and constant breeze. From time to time, we stopped to appreciate the scent of flowers and wild herbs, mixed by skillful alchemy with resin from the trees; the same alchemy that had suddenly made all our problems disappear. Nobody was

----

1   Our original Spanish lyrics were: Buenos días, Fuji. / Montañas verdes, / cielo azul. / Hola, monte Fuji. / A veces tímido, / te escondes entre las nubes. / Hola, Fuji. / La nieve blanca / es tu sombrero.

thinking about the stress of work anymore, or about the bitter aftertaste left from the academic year we'd just put an end to with this trip. All our anxiety and worries had dissolved thanks to the power of nature and fresh air. Without even knowing it, we were practicing the art of shinrin-yoku, literally translated as "forest bathing." The calm we had been unable to achieve during the year by means of relaxing massages, mindfulness sessions or even a sedative or two was now bestowed on us like a charm the moment we immersed ourselves in the greenery.

One of the conclusions we came to after living with the world's oldest people in Okinawa's village of centenaries was that to live surrounded by nature was key to understanding the secret of their longevity. Ogimi is in one of the densest regions of the Yanbaru[2] jungle that covers northern Okinawa. During our fieldwork, we asked one hundred old people about their diet, physical exercise, relationships with neighbors, and about *ikigai*: what it is that gets them out of bed and ready to live one more day. The nature that surrounds them plays a fundamental role in their physical, mental and spiritual well-being. As we mentioned at the end of our first book, in the 7th law of *ikigai*, despite the fact that most of us live in cities, we need to connect with nature on a regular basis, to go back and recharge our spiritual batteries.

Raimon, a famous singer-songwriter from Xativa, Valencia, sang the words of poet Joan Salvat-Papasseit: "when you forget where you come from, you forget who you are." In this book we'll explain how so many of the ailments afflicting city dwellers originate in our disconnect from nature. Being orphaned from the mother who gave us the breath of life,

---

2   Local word meaning "jungle of Okinawa".

spending our days, weeks and months surrounded by concrete blocks, separated from the natural habitat of our species is like being locked up in jail without realizing it. Dr. Shoma Morita, a pioneer of motivational therapy in the 1940s, began treatment by sending his patients to the forest, where he urged them to walk, chop firewood and rest among the trees. The results he obtained spectacularly surpassed the advances achieved in doctors' offices with medication. So is nature our best medicine? If it is, then how can we get back to nature and incorporate its essence into our busy urban lives?

An old Chinese proverb says: "Keep a green tree in your heart, and perhaps the singing bird will come." You don't need to live in the jungle of Okinawa or have a forest at your door, like our house in Hakone, to enjoy the healing powers of shinrin-yoku.

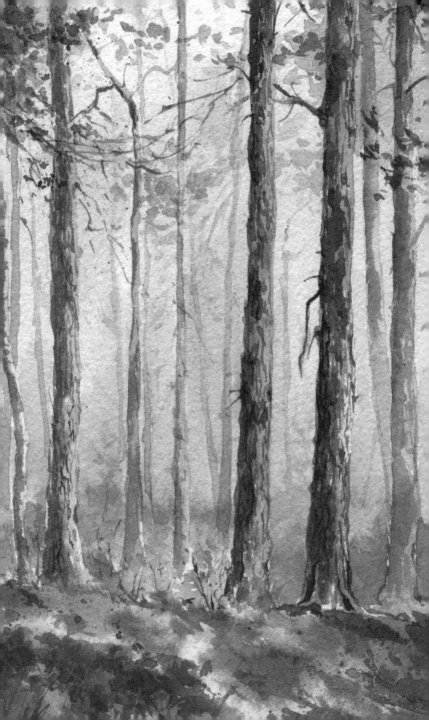

We've written this book with the idea of taking a leisurely, illuminating stroll together so that, wherever we are, we can make a green twig sprout in our lives and in our hearts.

—Héctor García and Francesc Miralles

What is *Shinrin-yoku*?

These days Japanese culture is primarily urban, yet more and more often you see groups, couples and even solo travelers heading into thickly wooded forests. Their pace is relaxed because they're not trying to get anywhere in particular. What they want to do is enjoy the healing and rejuvenating effects of *shinrin-yoku*, a term that was coined in 1982, when the director of the Japanese Forest Agency suggested that "bathing" in greenery provided very powerful health benefits to those who practiced it regularly. He was the first to suggest using this compound formed by the words *shinrin* "forests" and *yoku* "to bathe." And so began the use of this neologism, which has since become a world-wide trend.

SHINRIN-YOKU 森林海

森林 (forest)   海 (bathing or showering)

The use of nature as therapy was put to the test by the Japanese in the 1980s when they conducted revelatory studies showing that *shinrin-yoku* helps improve health even when people are temporarily unable to move. In one study, half of the patients in a hospital were placed in rooms having large windows with a forest view, while the other half had no windows. Patients having views onto greenery healed more quickly!

Growing interest on the part of health institutions sparked a multitude of scientific studies, which corroborated the Japanese Forest Agency's hypothesis that shinrin-yoku is a powerful therapy for relaxing the mind and reducing stress. In Part III of this book, we'll delve into the science to see the surprising results these studies have yielded. Dr. Morita knew only through intuition that nature healed his patients, but here in these pages we'll find out how.

The Magic of *Sakura*

Without doubt, the most beautiful time to visit Japan is during *sakura*, when cherry trees bloom in the spring and produce an explosion of white flowers to flood every heart. News programs include all kinds of forecasts for when this blossoming will begin in each city. Some companies even send an employee out to the nearest park in the middle of the night to stand guard under a tree, the goal being to save the spot so the work team can have a picnic if *sakura*'s flowers do indeed open.

When this happens, crowds pack the parks and tree-lined urban avenues. Couples take photographs with a sea of petals as background. It can transform the mood of an entire population, as serious, concentrated expressions make way for faces full of enthusiasm and permanent smiles. Everyone is suddenly more optimistic, as if the cherry blossoms were proof that life demands we live up to it by asking the best of us.

During *sakura*, people with life partners become more attentive, and many couples are seen having meals in restaurants near the trees. Those who are single at the time think about finding their soul mate, opening themselves up to love just in the same way the cherry trees show off their best-kept secret. Artists also bloom during *sakura*, becoming infected with the joy and creativity that fills the streets. New projects are undertaken to take advantage of the world as it shows its most delicate, dazzling and friendly face.

What happens at this time of year exemplifies to what extent trees can shape our state of mind, even in an urban setting. If this is what happens just by being on a boulevard or in a park lined with cherry trees, what effect will it have on our spirit to venture into a real forest, to walk in the silence of thousands of trees? This is what we'll be analyzing in this book, among many other things.

The Japanese and Their Love of Nature

Japanese people love the convenience of cities and the way they offer anything a consumer could possibly want, from Kobe meat (the best in the world) to cat cafes, but this culture's fascination with nature is pervasive. From *ikebana* and *haiku* to the philosophy of *wabi-sabi*—the art of imperfection that imitates nature, as we'll see later on—the natural world seeps into all aspects of daily life.

This becomes more patent, of course, the further we move away from cities and the closer we get to rural Japan. Towns aren't built around centers as they are in Europe; rather, their small houses are spread out here and there, wherever nature leaves them spaces, much like the shape of rice fields. In Part IV of this book, we'll discuss Japanese villages and their mysterious relationship with nature.

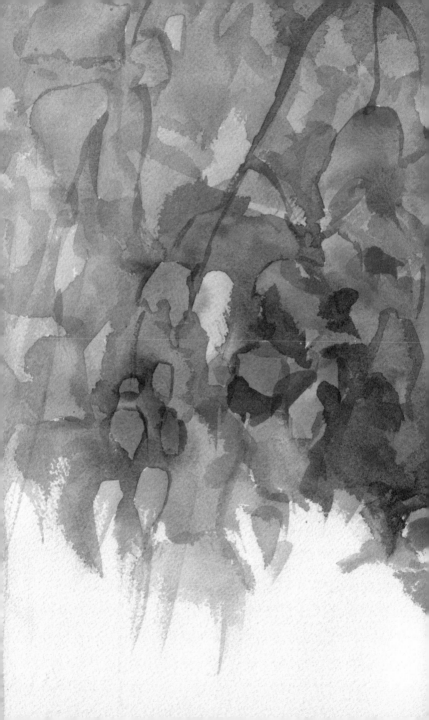

A GREEN HYMN

Love and the importance of nature in Japanese culture
are found even in the national anthem,
which includes this line:

"until the pebbles grow into boulders lush with moss."

This integration with nature is also apparent in the architecture of Buddhist temples and Shinto sanctuaries. Almost always surrounded by trees and built from wood, they form part of the natural landscape instead of dominating it. One of the most splendid statues of Buddha in all of Asia is found in Kamakura. If you turn right as you leave the station instead of taking the walking street, then continue down towards the sea, you'll find a peculiar building. A couple of balconies are missing from the first and second floors where space has been left for an enormous tree that looks like it's been there much longer than the building.

In many other places in Japan, it's clear that wise old trees take precedence over anything new and artificial. This could be where one of the secrets to shinrin-yoku resides. Let's dive right in.

The Healing Power of *Shinrin-yoku*
The benefits of shinrin-yoku aren't exclusive to walking in forests. We can experience them to a lesser degree in city parks, and even by having plants in the house to remind us of our connection to the earth.

More than thirty years after those first studies were made in the 1980s, the Japanese Society for Forest Medicine is providing opportunities for more than 10 million people to reconnect more often and more intensely with nature. This is true to such an extent that health insurance for many companies includes offering employees transportation and guides to green spaces outside the city. The aim is to reduce costly visits to doctors' offices, since no medicine has such broad applications as those offered by the fresh, lush embrace of trees.

HEALING EFFECTS OF *SHINRIN-YOKU*

Brain	• Helps produce more happiness hormones.
	• Mitigates aggression and sudden mood swings.
	• Helps repair damaged tissue.
	• Reduces the risk of dementia.
Eyes	• Relaxes and restores eyesight, which is greatly impaired by the constant use of screens on all our devices.
Heart	• Lowers blood pressure.
	• Slows heart rate.
Digestive System	• Taking a walk after a meal significantly improves digestion, even for people prone to constipation or diarrhea.
Immune System	• Naturally boosts our defenses, protecting us from disease.
Longevity	• As shown by the study done on *ikigai* in the village of centenaries, contact with nature increases life expectancy.

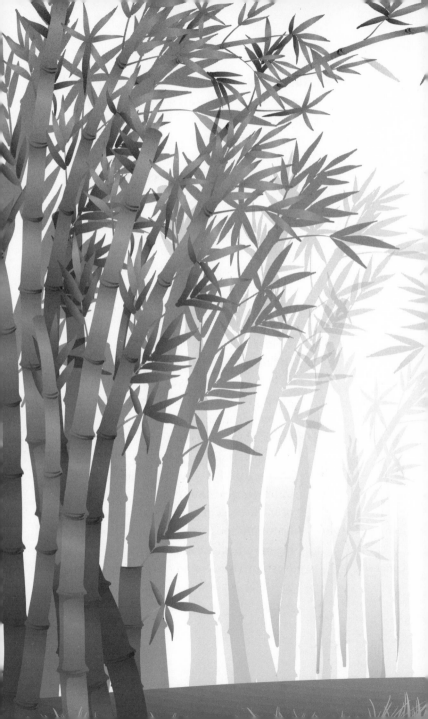

PART ONE

Paradise Lost

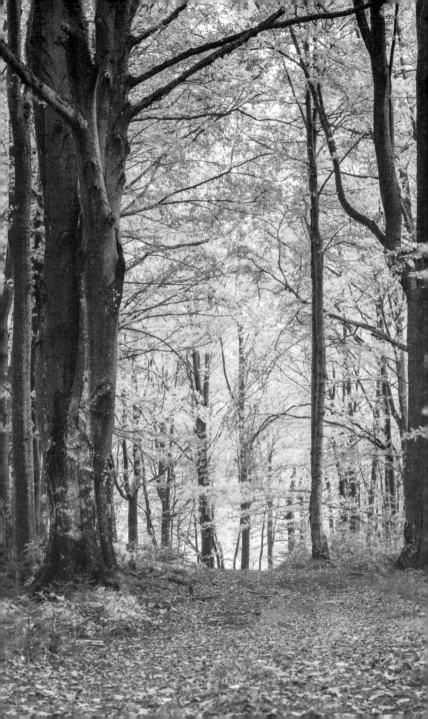

Our Disconnect with Nature

If we understand Genesis to be a narrative explaining the creation myth, in Spanish literary terms we might call it serendipity, seeing today's world and what it has become. Literary *serendipia* happens when a text describes something that didn't exist at the time it was written, but ends up existing later, as if an oracle had predicted it. In the novella *The Wreck of the Titan: Or, Futility*, for example, author Morgan Robertson narrated a scenario, fourteen years before the construction and sinking of the Titanic, that was full of similarities with the infamous transatlantic: the name and dimensions of the vessel, the collision with an iceberg, the captain's last name, and there being insufficient lifeboats for a ship full of multi-millionaires.

As regards the biblical account, the oracle is more allegorical than concrete—among other reasons, because thousands of years elapsed between the time of its writing and our time. Nevertheless, the message seems equally prophetic: modernity is the story of our expulsion from Paradise.

Living in Pipes

In the Garden of Eden, human beings lived in absolute harmony with nature and its cycles until they decided to fence in the fields and animals, build cities, and live in cabins that let in almost no sunlight. As "progress" arrived with the Industrial Revolution, the space in which people worked and lived was increasingly reduced until it's become the micro apartments being built these days in Tokyo, Manhattan and Hong Kong.

In the latter city, a lack of space and the high cost of housing have led to the sale of 10-square-meter apartments inside stackable concrete pipes. For the modest price of 15,000 euros—less than a car, according to the developer—you can live inside a pipe that's five meters long, two meters wide, and two meters high. As compressed as a spaceship, it has amenities that include a sofa-bed, a small bathroom with a shower, and the merest suggestion of a kitchen. Each end of the pipe has a glass door for getting in and out.

This is an extreme case, of course, but added to this unnatural act of living in a glorified "matchbox" is the fact that most people work in closed spaces and, at least in large cities, many millions of them travel underground between home and work. Consequently, a large part of the population rarely sees any sunlight or feels fresh air on their skin. If we're lucky, we might get to be outdoors for the few minutes it takes to walk home from the subway, the parking garage or the closest train station. Even so, we're still surrounded by buildings that make us feel like mice in a maze. No wonder, as we'll see in the next chapter, depression, anxiety and other stress-related illnesses feed off even those with enviable purchasing power.

Three Prices We Pay

Human beings are not meant to live like sewer rats. Like all other animals, we belong to our natural environment and, in order to stay balanced, we need to breathe clean, fresh air, feel the rich earth beneath our feet, and walk among the majestic trees that have always been part of our surroundings. Going back to Genesis, Adam and Eve let themselves be tempted by the serpent (a metaphor for ambition), leading to their expulsion from Paradise and their resulting pain, shame and labor. If we were to interpret biblical verses in the context of *serendipia*, or literary premonition, pain would be mortal stress, and worries would be the constant lack of time governing our lives far from Paradise. Shame would be another recognizable element of urban life, where the walls in our offices and homes separate us even from our own relatives, in contrast to our early communal life in the woods.

In Japan, the sense of privacy is so strong that people avoid looking each other in the eye, even when sharing a very tiny space like the subway. An executive could be looking at porn during rush hour yet remain confident that his fellow commuters won't even glance at what he's reading.

In regard to the way we understand labor, with work schedules, obligations, and pressures to reach goals, this is strictly an urban invention. Before we were expelled from Paradise, or expelled ourselves if belief in God is not the case, human beings were fluid in their hunting and gathering of food in accordance with seasons and life cycles. Clearly, we won't be returning to caves or going back to being nomadic hunters; however, it is within our power to once again benefit from a Garden of Eden-like well-being if we can just recapture the healing magic of nature, which is much closer than we think. This is what shinrin-yoku is all about.

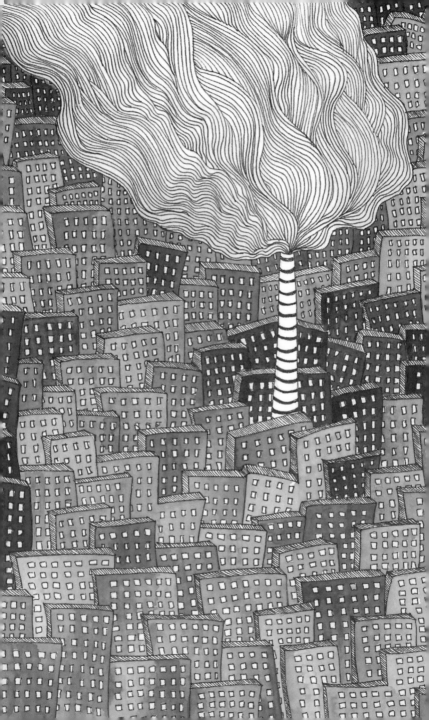

Stress in the City

The problem with cities isn't limited to the paradox of making us feel alone while surrounded by masses of people. More and more studies show the psychological damage caused by permanently turning our backs on nature in an overcrowded environment. In the words of Dr. Mazda Adli, psychiatrist and professor at the Humboldt University of Berlin: "if social density and social isolation occur at the same time and hit high-risk individuals, then city-stress related mental illness can often be the consequence." In a talk for TEDx-Berlin, he stated that our brains have not evolved sufficiently for us to live in overcrowded cities, and this has resulted in all kinds of anxiety-related disorders.

According to Dr. Adli, city living affects human health as much or more than global warming and, according to statistics, there is a 40% greater risk of suffering from depression in cities than in natural surroundings, and the chances of suffering from schizophrenia double. Where does this increase come from? One hypothesis is that a city's constant stimulation—noise in the streets, masses of people, advertizing everywhere—alters the way dopamine affects our bodies. This neurotransmitter is often related to pleasurable feelings and, in particular, relaxation, but it is essential to brain function on the whole. A shortage of dopamine affects all cognitive and emotional processes, and it's a problem often seen in people with psychological disorders.

As a group of Dutch medical researchers concluded: "life in the city may be part of the reason dopamine production begins to falter. Sustained stress has been shown to lead to this problem in many people."

An Eye-Opening Experiment

In a recent study, different groups of participants wore virtual reality headsets to walk around in the city, while others did so in predominantly natural surroundings. Different variables in participant physiology were measured during the experiment, clearly showing that getting around the city, even in a simulated world, causes stress to skyrocket, as well as negatively affecting mood. The visual and auditory stimulus overload, added to the presence of people everywhere, made participants feel overwhelmed, which unleashed negative emotions.

A MINDFULNESS EXERCISE

In an eight-week Mindfulness-Based Stress Reduction (MBSR) program, originally designed by Dr. Jon Kabat-Zinn, one of the exercises compares a calm stroll, such as one taken in a field, to the stress of walking through a city center. Participants begin walking in a full room of people who are walking quickly, changing direction every few steps and making an effort to not bump into each other. In the same way a calm stroll relaxes body and mind, when we find ourselves in the middle of a hurrying throng, stress immediately skyrockets, and some students even said they felt close to a panic attack.

This exercise is milder when done in a quiet classroom, however, than it would be on the street where there would also be noise (among other stimuli) as well as the fact that many people don't see others and may even bump into them because they march along stressed out and texting on their phones.

In major cities, a shortage of space has led to thousands of skyscrapers also being built for housing. Studies on the effect of living in these high-rises, as compared to living in houses or low-rise buildings, have shown that there are increased cases of stress, neuroses and even developmental problems in children.

In an article for *The Guardian*, Joey Gardiner, a journalist specializing in architecture, mentions the research done by professor Colin Ellard, who, while walking past the huge buildings in downtown Toronto, experienced a moment of insight: "I was struck by how dark, sombre and sad these new urban canyons made me feel."

A University of Waterloo neuroscientist who specializes in the impact of places on the brain and body, Ellard wondered if the same thing happened to other people. Using the virtual reality experiments we mentioned earlier, he discovered that being surrounded by tall buildings had a substantial negative impact on mood. This clashes with the commercial reality of cities like London, where four hundred skyscrapers are under construction. How can we live this way without compromising our physical and mental health? Once again, getting back in touch with nature by regularly "bathing in forests" is the answer.

COUNTRY LIVING

Low risk of mental illness.

Silence or the sounds of nature.

Fewer relationships, but deeper social connections.

Abundance of green.[3]

Curved, irregular lines.

Low levels of cortisol and many other stress markers.

CITY LIVING

Greater risk of mental illness.

Noise and tension.

Connecting with multitudes, but surrounded by strangers.

Lack of the color green and predominance of gray.

Straight lines and edges.[4]

High cortisol (stress hormone) levels.

---

3 Evidence from studies on the benefits of the color green indicates that having some plants or even just posters with green in them in the office reduces stress in employees.

4 Edges and straight lines seem threatening to us because we unconsciously see them as unnatural, as something that might be dangerous or harmful.

Blue Zones, Green Cities

Blue Zones offer substantial proof of the health benefits from contact with nature. These five places, home to the longest-living people in the world, are all relatively undeveloped and in natural environments. We visited one of them when we were writing *Ikigai*. The so-called "Village of Centenaries" is in northern Okinawa, and its residents live surrounded by the jungle and the sea.

The four other Blue Zones are also places in the country where residents are in constant contact with greenery. In the Nuoro and Ogliastra provinces of Sardinia, there are many small villages where 100-year-old residents walk back and forth over the countryside, and even some who still shepherd their flocks of sheep. Loma Linda in California is another one of the Blue Zones. With a population of less than 20,000 inhabitants, close ties are maintained through neighborhood associations, and residents are surrounded by forests and green spaces dotted here and there with small houses.

The peninsula of Nicoya, in Costa Rica, is another place where inhabitants practically live in the jungle, much like the Japanese of northern Okinawa. And, finally, the fifth Blue Zone is Ikaria, in Greece. This mountainous island has small villages scattered throughout the forests but with views to the sea, and a total population of less than 10,000 people.

In addition to the direct benefits of shinrin-yoku these people enjoy, another important factor in their longevity is the food they consume, which they grow themselves.

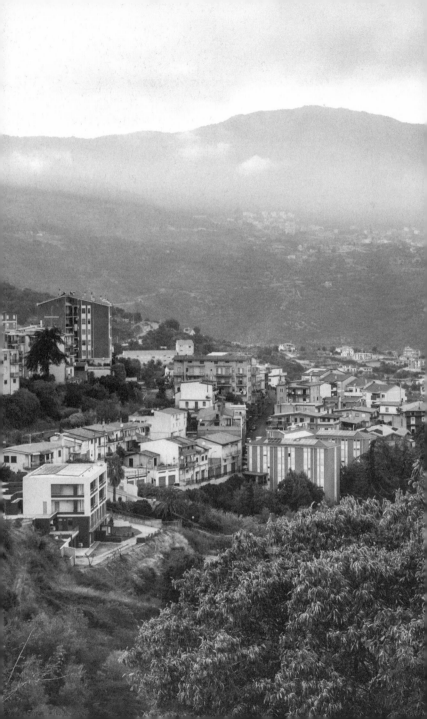

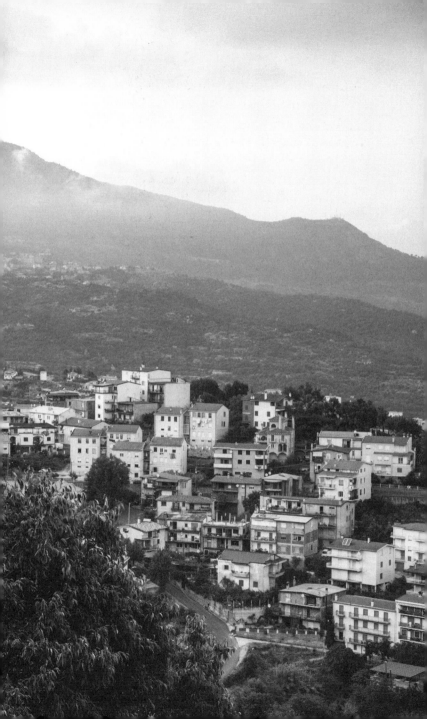

Cities of the Future

Even though only a tiny part of the world's population lives in Blue Zones, urban planners are increasingly conscious of the need to integrate nature with cities. Japan is a good example of this. Although Tokyo is a megalopolis with thousands of skyscrapers, almost no one lives in its vertical spaces. The majority of inhabitants live far from these centers, many in small houses on the outskirts of the city. As soon as you leave the main train stations, you see streets start to curve, and you get the feeling that the parks are like magnetic fields around which everything else has been built.

The residential neighborhoods of Setagaya-ku, Nakano-ku and Bunkyo-ku are perfect examples of this phenomenon in Tokyo. You can't walk five minutes from house to house before you come across a temple surrounded by trees, or a garden that makes you forget you're in a huge city. Maybe that's why these are the places where many of the main characters in Murakami novels roam.

Aerial views of Tokyo show a city with fractal, irregular shapes highlighted by three major green spaces: the Imperial Palace, Yoyogi Park, and the gardens of Shinjuku Gyoen. From the top of a skyscraper in Tokyo, all around us we see one of the largest conurbations in the world, yet ever on the horizon, marking the boundaries of the Kanto region, are the green mountains of Tanzawa and Okutama and, behind them, majestic Mount Fuji keeps watch over it all. Japanese cities are gigantic, but they rarely expand into the mountains. Instead, they advance towards the sea, where artificial islands are built to be the site for future airports and more housing.

In many European cities, where demographic pressure isn't quite so immediate, urban-planning restrictions are being established to keep cities on a more human scale, and so escape the alienation mentioned by the professor from Toronto. For example, Barcelona does not permit construction of skyscrapers outside the business district. Buildings are restricted to a maximum of eight floors, and this limit is reduced by half in the walkable (and hipster) neighborhood of Gracia. In regard to this city, architect Antoni Gaudí was a pioneer in applying the language of nature to his buildings. Expanding on his idea that "originality consists in returning to the origin," the creator of the Sagrada Familia noted that "the straight line belongs to Man, the curved line to God." Because a straight line is not nature's way, as we will see when we get into *wabi-sabi*, everything in structures like Güell Park is organic and curvilinear, in homage to all that awaits us beyond the city limits.

A Strong and Beautiful Tree

No matter where we live, in the deepest recesses of every human being lies a desire to reconnect with nature. To prove it, just look at children in the city. Though they've grown up among concrete blocks, when they go out to the countryside and see a real live tree, their natural impulse is to climb it. We've all fantasized as children about having a tree house all our own, which is something more and more green hotels are catering to. Going to sleep to the gentle rush of wind through trees, and waking a few feet from birdsong is, without doubt, an illuminating experience.

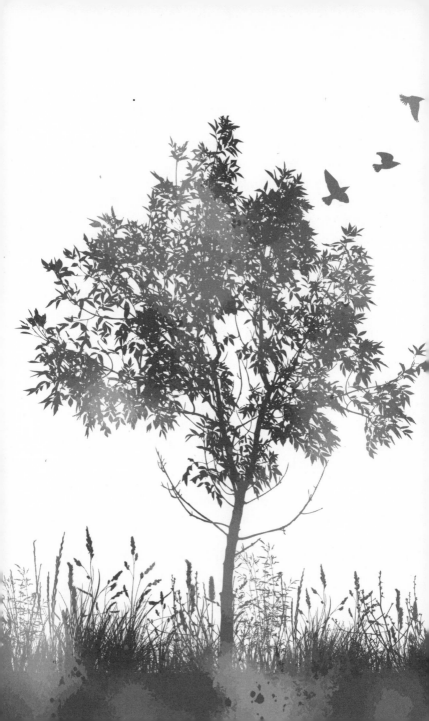

Soundtrack for the Soul

"As a lifelong birder I've always had birdsong as a natural soundtrack to my life and believe it's good for the mind and soul. Birdsong gets us closer to nature and links people to places and memories in a way that few other sounds can. [...] It's a simple pleasure that most of us can enjoy, even if we live in towns and cities."

—Peter Brash, ecologist at the UK's National Trust

Since we can't indulge in such bucolic vacations, this book will show us how to incorporate "green bathing" into our daily lives. But before we begin our practice, the following chapters will tell us why trees have been so inspirational to all spiritual traditions.

Hermann Hesse revered them as sacred in *Wandering*, a collection of contemplative texts from 1920, accompanied in the original by thirteen watercolor landscapes: "For me, trees have always been the most penetrating preachers. I revere them when they live in tribes and families, in forests and groves. And even more I revere them when they stand alone. They are like lonely persons. Not like hermits who have stolen away out of some weakness, but like great, solitary men, like Beethoven and Nietzsche. In their highest boughs the world rustles, their roots rest in infinity; but they do not lose themselves there, they struggle with all the force of their lives for one thing only: to fulfill themselves according to their own laws, to build up their own form, to represent themselves. Nothing is holier, nothing is more exemplary than a beautiful, strong tree."

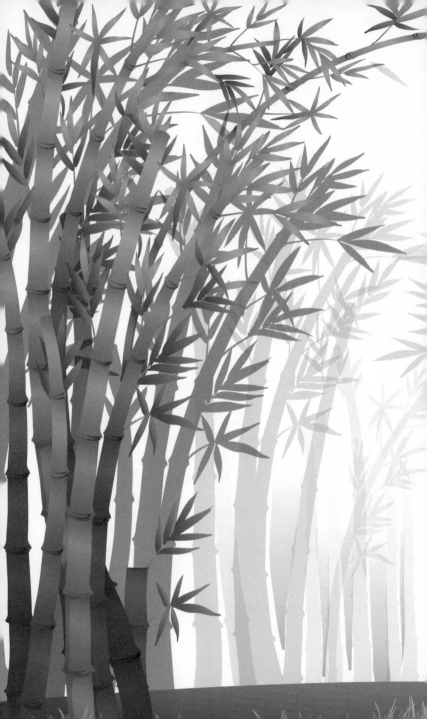

PART TWO

Return to the
Garden of Eden

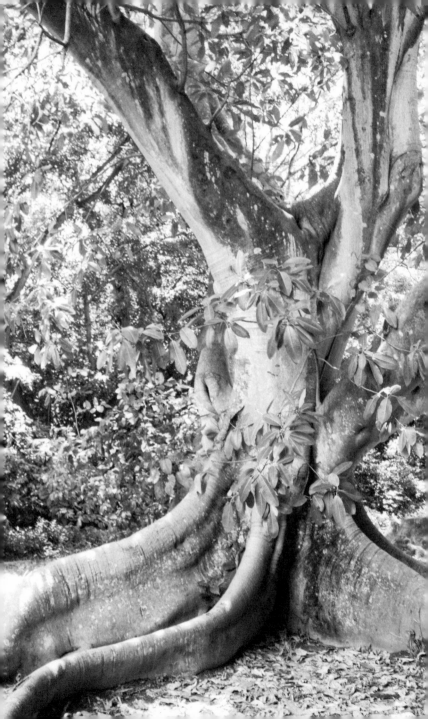

The Bodhi Tree

The life of Siddhartha Gautama bears out Hermann Hesse's closing thought in the last chapter of Part I. After a long life of pilgrimage, full of hardship and sacrifice, Buddha attained enlightenment by sitting under the shade of a tree. Born a prince, he had fled the palace after seeing an old man, a sick man and a dead man, and went in search of the reason behind human suffering, and a possible solution to it. The ascetic's rigorous fasting gave him no answers, nor did the many other exercises in self-mortification he practiced on his journey along with other seekers. Then he found his defining inspiration in a tree. Upon seeing a hardy fig tree, Siddhartha decided to sit under it and vowed he would not get up until he discovered the truth about human suffering.

Nature's Temple of Enlightenment

Legend has it that Siddhartha Gautama sat in the shade of the fig tree for a total of seven weeks. When a terrible storm broke, Mucalinda, King of the Serpents, emerged from beneath the roots and wrapped itself around Siddhartha's entire body like a wetsuit to protect him from the storm. Under this tree he attained full awakening (bodhi) and so became the Buddha. What he had not managed to learn in any human temple, from any teacher or scholar, he learned in the silence of the tree that had been his inspiration in discovering the essence of Buddhism: human suffering is caused by desire, the desire to have new things as well as to keep what we already have—attachment. We cling to it all in a world which is itself impermanent (everything changes, dies and passes on). This is why we experience the fear of loss. If we free ourselves from all desire, from all attachment, and embrace the present, then suffering stops.

Buddha so was grateful to that tree for having brought him enlightenment that it is said he spent an entire week looking at the fig tree without blinking even once. The Bodhi Tree became a pilgrimage site from that very moment, and following the departure of the illuminated one, its fame continued to grow.

Among its devotees, King Asoka (304-232 BCE), considered to be the founder of India, went every year to pay tribute to the sacred fig tree, even paying for a festival in its honor. This devotion to the tree made his wife jealous. Once the royal scepter was in her hands, she gave orders to have the tree killed using poisonous thorns, but the faithful planted a shoot from the original fig tree in the same place. Today it continues to thrive in the city of Bodh Gaya, in northwest India, where it is currently sheltered within the imposing Mahabodhi Temple ("Great Awakening" in Sanskrit) and is visited by thousands of pilgrims each year. Silence is demanded when pilgrims approach the fig tree, as if twenty-five hundred years later, Siddartha Gautama were still immersed in meditation.

OTHER TREES WORTH VISITING

1. *The Tree of Life.* In the middle of the Bahrain Desert, this four-hundred-year-old acacia is the most isolated tree in the world. There is not a single drop of water to be found for many kilometers in any direction, which makes its survival a complete enigma. Some local mystics insist that its origins go back to the Garden of Eden.

2. *General Sherman.* Sequoia National Park, California. This tree has the greatest biomass in the world. Calculated to be two thousand years old, its base has a diameter of eleven meters, or thirty-six and a half feet.

3. Árbol de Tule, or *Tree of Tule.* This Montezuma cypress has the stoutest trunk in the world. With a forty-two meter (almost 140 ft.) diameter, it takes thirty people holding hands to hug it, and it can give shade to five hundred people.

Living Examples

Buddha's colorful history, however, is not unique. Since the beginning of civilization, mystics have looked to forests in search of inspiration. In the case of meditators, the reason is obvious: trees embody the position and essence of the act of contemplation. Firmly seated on the ground, like a yogi who never abandons his posture until the session is over, the trunk is the meditator's back, held straight and in a dignified position, and the treetop is his head. While meditating, the thoughts running through our mind could be in the hundreds or thousands, as many as there are leaves in a tree stirred by the breeze, but instead of judging them, holding onto them or rejecting them, we let them go. They are just thoughts; leaves ruffled by the wind. They have nothing to do with the steady heart of the contemplative person who, like a tree, forms a bridge between the depths of the earth and the immensity of the heavens. The living example of serenity and majesty afforded us by trees serves as an invitation to sit in their shade, an invitation extended to readers (can there be anything more delightful than sitting under a tree and reading a good book?), writers, artists, philosophers and scientists. It's no coincidence that one of the most relevant discoveries in the history of science, Newton's Law of Gravity, took place, as legend has it, under an apple tree.

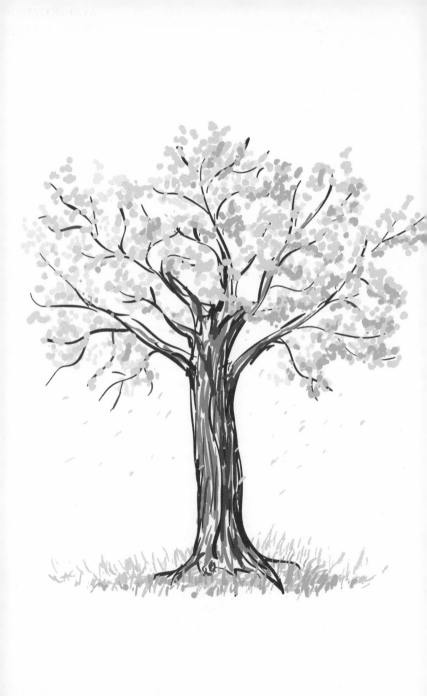

Hanasaka Jiisan—The Old Man Who Made the Dead Trees Blossom

A traditional Japanese story tells the tale of an elderly couple who never had children. They lived a quiet life with their dog in the mountains. One morning, the dog began digging behind the house next to a fig tree, and barked to attract its masters' attention. It had uncovered a chest full of gold coins!

A neighbor who heard about the discovery, thinking the dog had special powers, asked to borrow the animal. Seeing that the dog, after many unfruitful attempts, didn't unearth anything of value, he grew angry. So filled with rage was he that instead of giving the dog back to the couple, the neighbor killed it and buried it beside the same fig tree where the treasure had been unearthed.

The old couple were miserable about all that had happened, and they missed their pet so much that they dreamt of it often. In one of the dreams, the dog said to its master, who was called Hanasaka: "You must cut down the fig tree and use the wood to carve a mallet for pounding rice into paste."

When he woke up, he talked to his wife about the strange request and, though they were sorry about cutting down the tree, they decided to fulfill their good friend's wishes. Once the mallet had been carved from the chopped fig tree, they used it to pound and knead the rice, just as the animal had asked, and then they realized something wonderful was happening. Each time the mallet struck, grains of rice turned into gold dust.

The news reached that same neighbor, who once again went to the old couples' house and asked to borrow the mallet.

Despite what had happened to their dog, and because they were kind, the old couple agreed once more. Convinced that he would be able to amass a huge fortune in gold from the lowly rice, the neighbor began to pound the grains with the mallet, but he flew into a fury when he saw that what had been food from his pantry was turning into rotten berries. He went to give the mallet back to old couple, and demanded all sorts of explanations from them. To appease the neighbor's anger, they finally decided to burn the mallet right in front of him.

That night, the dog again appeared to its master in a dream and said: "As soon as you can, gather up the ashes of the mallet and scatter them near the cherry trees."

When the old couple rose, they immediately went to scatter the ashes by the cherry trees, just as the dog had asked. Their eyes lit up when they saw the trees burst into bloom, even though spring was still far off. In just a few hours, the cherry trees on the mountain and on the roads to the village were all more beautiful than ever, festooned with *sakura*. Suffused with happiness, the old couple scattered some of ashes at the foot of a few cherry trees that had died a long time before, and these also came back to life and were full of flowers.

When the *daimio* (feudal lord) journeyed through that land, he was filled with wonder at what he saw. Upon learning it was the elderly couple who had worked the miracle, he gave them valuable gifts as a reward.

Wild with envy, the neighbor ran to grab a handful of ashes. He also scattered them next to a dead tree to try to impress the *daimio* and receive gifts. But a gust of wind lifted the ashes, blowing them into the eyes of the feudal lord and blinding him. He sentenced the neighbor to prison.

Nature's Retribution

This tale has the surreal, fanciful character of many Japanese stories, but it contains key elements to help us understand the essence of shinrin-yoku. In nature, everything is transformed to make room for something better. The dead dog becomes a wise night counselor. The fig tree becomes a spirit able to turn rice into gold. Its ashes become fertilizer bringing the trees back to life as if by magic.

In the same way, people walking in the forest will come out transformed. They'll come back from their excursion with a treasure worth much more than the gold in the story: serenity in their souls, harmony, mental balance, and new ideas for making any necessary changes in their lives. Yet in order for this to happen, there must be a willingness to listen to nature. In the story, the neighbor never receives anything of value because he is guided only by greed and a thirst for artificial wealth. The dog's masters, on the other hand, do listen to nature, and that's why good fortune accompanies them. The tale of *Hanasaka Jiisan*,[5] as it is known in Japan, is full of the Japanese mythology we see in Studio Ghibli films: trees with wonderful attributes, talking animals and Shinto spirits. In short, an interconnectedness among all living beings.

Getting back to shinrin-yoku, the message is clear. Everything we give to nature when we devote our time, energy and attention to it is given back to us in abundance in the form of riches such as health, serenity and inspiration.

---

5 In English, "The Old Man Who Made Flowers Blossom".

The Sages of the Bamboo Grove

Chinese tradition encourages a close relationship between connecting with nature and cultivating a spiritual life. The best example of this is the Seven Sages (or Worthies) of the Bamboo Grove, a group of poets, artists and philosophers from the third century CE. They gathered under a bamboo grove to chat, compose and recite poetry while enjoying drink and music. Far from the intrigues of the Court during the Three Kingdoms period, their natural refuge was in Henan province, near the home of one of them, Xi Kang, whose relationship with another member of the group, Ruan Ji, was described as being "stronger than metal and fragrant as orchids."

This enlightened group of Taoists enjoyed the simple life in the midst of nature. Fleeing the politics of the time, they created a haven of art and free thought in the shade of the tall bamboo stalks. It is said that the fellowship among these seven men was such that they could communicate without saying a word, using only subtle gestures or a smile.

POEMS FROM MY HEART

Ruan Ji was famous for eight poems he wrote criticizing
the frivolous, superficial life in the city at the time,
compared to the pure, serene life in the forest.
This is one of them:

And by the river one hears decadent songs.
These idle, empty-headed youths,
slaves to fashion and fantasy,
always in search of the short cut
leading them to pleasure.

I see no one wanting to rise before the sun
or take their walking stick to the forest.
To follow the recipe for a long life
is what calms the turmoil in my heart.[6]

Philosophy in the Forest

The Seven Sages, in addition to being scholars in different disciplines, practiced the art of *qingtan*, which is translated from the Chinese as "pure conversation." It involved debating freely on any aesthetic, philosophical or metaphysical subject, in a similar way to classical Greek philosophers. Witty phrases that analyzed reality or invented definitions were bandied about. They explored the meaning of life, the art of living, and the feelings that make us human.

Qingtan survived the Seven Sages of the bamboo grove and continued to be practiced by intellectual elites in the centuries that followed. Some of these conversations and reflections were collected in the 5th-century anthology *Shishuo Xinyu* by Liu Yiqinq.

Chinese culture was a pioneer in holding spiritual retreats in the midst of nature.

In Harmony with Tao

The era in which the Seven Sages lived was dominated by a dynasty with a Confucian ethic, which caused these free spirits to be viewed with suspicion by the Court. Instead of following the established morals and norms, they all wanted to become one with the Tao, the natural pulse of life. They believed that people who live in harmony with nature, far from the city's artifice, will also be at peace with themselves.

....
6 Translator note: Translated into English from the Spanish.

In addition to being the mystics and Bohemians of their era, some of these sages were said to be initiated in the secrets of alchemy, thanks to their observations of nature. Much like the cynical Greeks, the Sages of the Bamboo Grove were known for being eccentric, even crazy buffoons. They were capable of debating philosophy and art for hours on end, reciting poetry and playing delicate musical pieces, but they could also go crazy on great drunken binges that ended with them dancing naked in the forest.

Their life's motto was so-called *feng lin* or, in English, "to depart from convention." A standout among them was Liu Ling, who was very fond of alcohol and not at all fond of clothes. It's said that on one occasion a visitor arrived wanting to see him, and was astonished to find him completely naked. On noticing his visitor's surprise, the sage Taoist spat out:

"I consider the universe to be my home and my house to be my clothing. So get out of my pants!"

Trees of the Celtic Forest

Ancient Celts also believed the forest to be the center of their universe. For them, life took place under the spreading branches of trees, on the leaf-covered paths they shared with animals and the legendary creatures of their beliefs. They were at home in the forests where they found food, heat in winter and wood for their houses and boats, but also shelter for their spirits.

Trees were at the core of their mythology and were considered sacred as a result of generations observing and learning their cycles and vital phenomena. Through intermediaries such as druids or priests, the Celts conversed with nature and made appeals to the gods to ask for their favor. In fact, the proximity of these men and women to trees was such that they tended to live near them, and barely went near the towns. These European sages of the forest, like Merlin, acted as real guides for their communities, thanks to their mystical and medical knowledge, and so held quite high positions in the hierarchies of their towns and villages.

The Three Dimensions of the Tree of Life

Ancient Celtic wisdom divides trees into three parts, all having clear symbolic content. The first is the trunk, the material from which firewood is obtained for warmth, and food for survival. The second part is in the roots, which are secret because they're hidden in the earth. They represent all the wisdom that nature can hold. The third and last part is the crown of the tree, which looks towards the sky at something beyond what is purely human.

Every tree, therefore, embodies these three dimensions of human beings:

- Our capacity to keep warm and care for our own body, as well as those of our loved ones.
- The wisdom that allows us to get the most out of life, as well as the secrets of nature and human existence.
- The desire to rise above our daily lives and seek meaning and transcendence beyond ourselves.

This triple cosmology is represented by the Tree of Life, an image still found today in pins, pendants and all kinds of Celtic-inspired ornaments.

The Tree of Life unites heaven and earth through the bark of the tree, illustrating these three dimensions of human beings.

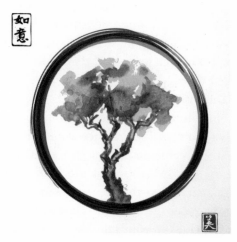

The Forest as Rite of Passage

As with Shinto temples, the temples of the Celts were sacred groves. Some were prohibited to the uninitiated, and magical properties were attributed to them. They are found over a large stretch of Northern Europe, an area that was dominated by Celts until being invaded by Roman and Germanic tribes.

The sacred grove was a place for venerating the gods that were related to trees and nature. Fairies and fabulous creatures were part of Celtic mythology, and were always willing to make appearances in the thickly wooded forests. These same groves were the settings for Celtic myths like Finn McCool, and the adventures of Cú Chulainn on his journey to Scathach.

Known as the Irish Achilles by virtue of his exploits, Cú Chulainn aspired to train as a hero to attract the attention of Emer, the most beautiful young woman in Ulster. In order to reach the mythical Scathach in the Fortress of Shadows and be taught by her, he had to cross deep, untamed forests that, according to legend, swallowed all who ventured to enter.

The mythology of the "dark forest" continues to resonate today. We can see it in such recent series as the youth-oriented *Stranger Things*, where the trunk of a tree (as in *Alice in Wonderland*) is the gateway to a full world of dangers requiring the utmost bravery of its protagonists.

The forest as a "rite of passage" from childhood to adulthood is a part of many civilizations. In the traditional cultures of Africa or the Amazon, teenagers had to go into the jungle and survive several days by hunting and defending themselves from wild animals. After passing this test, which had the forest as a threshold, they returned as empowered men to take on the challenges of adult life.

Our urban lives are so far removed from forests that returning to them becomes another extraordinary adventure which, though on a much smaller scale, will always leave us transformed.

TREE THERAPY: HUG A TREE

Tree hugging, practiced since the time of the Druids and revived by Wicca practitioners, is now recognized as tree therapy, or forest therapy. We know, for instance, that koalas hug eucalyptus and acacia trees to cool off during Australia's sweltering summers. They don't need to get down as often to drink water, so there's less risk of running into predators. Human beings, on the other hand, are potentially our own predators.

In his book *Blinded by Science*, Matthew Silverstone discusses studies that show how hugging trees relieves anxiety and helps us to free ourselves of negative thoughts. According to Silverstone, the benefits have to do with the almost imperceptible vibrations given off by tree trunks. We don't notice them consciously, but our organism does, and so manages to regain its balance by taking medicine directly from nature, with no prescriptions or pills.

Wicca: Modern Witchcraft

The Celtic worship of trees has survived to the present day under a neo-pagan religion that emerged in mid-20th century England with Gerald Gardner as its principal exponent. The son of a family that imported hardwood from Borneo and Malaysia, Gardner lived in Asia for much of his life. In 1936 he decided to return to England, where, being convinced of the great benefits of sunbathing, he embraced nudism, and began taking an interest in Celtic magic.

After being initiated by the witch Dorothy Clutterbuck, he began writing treatises and collaborating with pagan priestesses like Doreen Valiente. Together they created the rituals for a new religion called Wicca, an Old English word for "witch." When he died, in 1964, this belief system that draws from Celtic magic spread all over the world. In fact, the 13 Principles of Wiccan belief were drafted ten years later by the Council of American Witches. These are the first two:

1. We practice rites to attune ourselves with the natural rhythm of life forces marked by the phases of the Moon and the seasonal Quarters and Cross Quarters.

2. We recognize that our intelligence gives us a unique responsibility toward our environment. We seek to live in harmony with Nature, in ecological balance offering fulfillment to life and consciousness within an evolution-ary concept.

   Although a note clarifies that Wicca practitioners don't reject conventional medical treatment, the last principle connects with the therapeutic essence of shinrin-yoku:

3. We believe that we should seek within Nature that which is contributory to our health and well-being.

Their beliefs are based on dual divinity, a goddess and a god, representing different elements of nature, in accordance with the different schools of Wicca. For the followers of eclectic Wicca, the goddess is the moon and sea, whereas the god is the forests and animals. The followers of this neo-pagan religion believe we have deep ties to nature and all other living beings, who are our brothers and sisters. In the words of Doreen Valiente, "Magic, indeed, is all around us, in stones, flowers, stars, the dawn wind and the sunset cloud; all we need is the ability to see and understand."

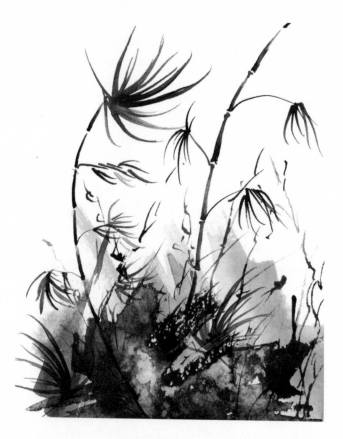

Thoreau's Adventure

Now that we've explored the magic in forests as understood by various spiritual traditions, let's move on to the modern world. Who hasn't sometimes thought of leaving everything behind and heading off to a cabin in the woods? The popular Spanish expression "cómprate un bosque y piérdete" (make like a tree and leave, but literally "buy a forest and get lost") plays with this idea. The American philosopher and pioneer in civil disobedience, Henry David Thoreau, did just that in the 19th century and documented it all. Thoreau was a great student of natural history and everything that had to do with it. He closely followed everything Darwin published after his voyage on the Beagle. Nevertheless, the big change in his life came with the challenge and experience he recorded in his diary, *Walden; or, Life in the Forest*.

Two years, Two Months and Two Days
Having had enough of the society of his time, he decided to leave his home in Concord and go live in a cabin in the woods for a particular period of time: two years, two months and two days.

WHERE I LIVED, AND WHAT I LIVED FOR

"I went to the woods because I wished to live deliberately, to front only the essential facts of life, and see if I could not learn what it had to teach, and not, when I came to die, discover that I had not lived. I did not wish to live what was not life, living is so dear; nor did I wish to practise resignation, unless it was quite necessary. I wanted to live deep and suck out all

> the marrow of life, to live so sturdily and Spartan-like as to put to rout all that was not life..."
>
> —Henry David Thoreau

Thoreau built his own cabin near Walden Pond, recycling parts from a deconstructed shed, as well as second-hand windows and roof shingles. But we mustn't imagine his experience as being a true ascetic retreat, either. Almost every day he walked to Concord, a highly relevant historical place that, together with neighboring Lexington, was where America's Revolutionary War began. There he bought the newspaper, got food and even visited relatives.

Thoreau's cabin saw no shortage of visitors, either. One of the most prominent figures he chatted with during his experiment in living in nature by Walden Pond was Nathaniel Hawthorne, one of the most renowned novelists of the time. Yet despite these details, which may be somewhat demystifying, Thoreau's book begins with the following words:

> When I wrote the following pages, or rather the bulk of them, I lived alone, in the woods, a mile from any neighbor, in a house which I had built myself, on the shore of Walden Pond, in Concord, Massachusetts, and earned my living by the labor of my hands only. I lived there two years and two months. At present I am a sojourner in civilized life again.

After living that long in nature, Thoreau felt transformed by the contemplative existence he experienced, with occasional exceptions, in the solitude of the woods. But what was he trying to do with this experiment? Essentially, he wanted to prove that life in natural surroundings provides human beings with everything they need: true freedom and self-knowledge. After the retreat that led him to stay in the small cabin, Thoreau felt he had to go back to the city. What he learned in the forest, however, would stay with him for the rest of his life.

Walking in the Woods

The American philosopher never stopped turning to nature and reflecting on it. The lecture-turned-essay he wrote following his time at Walden, which was published posthumously as *Walking*, begins with this firm declaration of intent:

> I wish to speak a word for Nature, for absolute Freedom and Wildness, as contrasted with a freedom and culture merely civil,—to regard man as an inhabitant, or a part and parcel of Nature, rather than a member of society.

Nature is the true refuge of man, and this is why Thoreau defends returning to the place where life began thousands of years ago. It's about closing the circle by returning to the woods because it is there, in the open air, with just the treetops and the sky above us, where we gain true freedom of spirit, something we can't get from the comforts of home. In this text, the author of *Walden* makes some interesting points when he talks about the benefits of walking, though not on an urban surface in a concrete labyrinth, but in the lushness of the forest. In fact, he explains how, on many occasions, it ends up happening automatically:

> When we walk, we naturally go to the fields and woods: what would become of us, if we walked only in a garden or a mall? [...] Of course it is of no use to direct our steps to the

woods, if they do not carry us thither. I am alarmed when it happens that I have walked a mile into the woods bodily, without getting there in spirit.

In my afternoon walk I would fain forget all my morning occupations and my obligations to society. But it sometimes happens that I cannot easily shake off the village. The thought of some work will run in my head and I am not where my body is—I am out of my senses. In my walks I would fain return to my senses.

What business have I in the woods, if I am thinking of something out of the woods? I suspect myself, and cannot help a shudder when I find myself so implicated even in what are called good works—for this may sometimes happen.

Without knowing it, Thoreau was writing a user's manual for shinrin-yoku, which we'll see how to practice in Part V of this book. He posits that roads are made for getting from one place to another quickly, not for sauntering in no particular direction. For that, we already have something growing freely, with earth instead of asphalt under it. Because, as one of Thoreau's own quotes goes: "There are moments when all anxiety and stated toil are becalmed in the infinite leisure and repose of nature."

The Root of All Ills

For Thoreau, the illnesses of the body and spirit of modern human beings have their origin in the unnatural custom of closing ourselves up behind four walls, and leaving only to go into the city to run quick errands and then return to our confinement. In his own words:

I, who cannot stay in my chamber for a single day without acquiring some rust, and when sometimes I have stolen forth for a walk at the eleventh hour, or four o'clock in the afternoon, too late to redeem the day, when the shades of night were already beginning to be mingled with the daylight, have felt as if I had committed some sin to be atoned for,—I confess that I am astonished at the power of endurance, to say nothing of the moral insensibility, of my neighbors who confine themselves to shops and offices the whole day for weeks and months, aye, and years almost together. [...] How womankind, who are confined to the house still more than men, stand it I do not know; but I have ground to suspect that most of them do not STAND it at all.

Even though we may not have hours to take a walk every day like this 19th-century thinker did, it's important to be aware of what our natural scenario is, so we can return to it at least once a week. Just as believers periodically attend the house of God, if we're aware of what our soul needs, then we will need to return to the house of human beings, in fact, of every living being: nature.

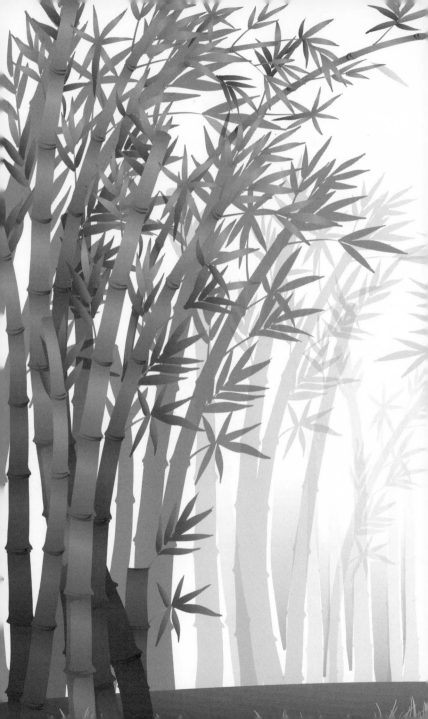

PART THREE

The Science of *Shinrin-Yoku*

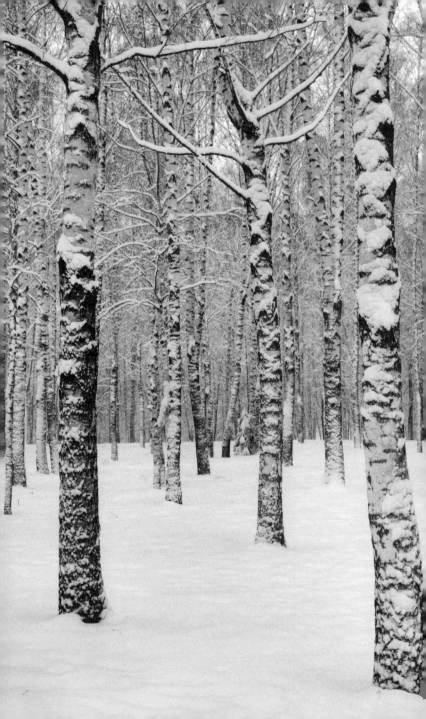

What Doesn't Kill Us Makes Us Stronger

The title for this chapter comes from a quote by Friedrich Nietzsche and, as we will see in a moment, it has a surprising amount to do with the science behind shinrin-yoku.

Those of us who are fans of *Dragon Ball* are well aware of the power of senzu, or magic beans. When a *saiyan* is so wounded as to be on the brink of death but takes a magic bean, he gets better and becomes more powerful than he was originally. Being hurt in small doses benefits the *saiyan* in *Dragon Ball* because its unleashes their power. Neither fantasy nor philosopher's aphorism, the scientific grounds on which shinrin-yoku works is based on the same principle. In this chapter we will learn how nature makes us stronger by hurting us silently and in small doses.

From Tradition to Science

We may be tempted to think that all belief based on tradition is the antithesis of science, but in fact they often go hand in hand. For most of history, people have used "non-scientific" strategies to survive. After all, when we interact with the world, we are always calibrating what we do by "trial and error," which is the basis of science. As we go along trying one thing or another, we become aware of what works and what doesn't. Some traditions die while others prove themselves useful to our survival. For thousands of years in traditional medicine, if one potion didn't cure us, we died; if another one worked, we continued to use it. It wasn't until the last few centuries that science had the means to conduct research on what we intuitively knew thanks to tradition. And we will be discussing this in relation to the healing power of forests.

In the early part of the 20th century, Dr. Shoma Morita[7] took his patients for walks in the forest and had them cut firewood every day, aware that the regenerative capacity of nature on body and soul is greater than many medications. If he'd had access to the data we now have available, and which we share here in Part III, he'd have seen his intuitions confirmed.

In fact, the Japanese have used nature as treatment for thousands of years. Shinto places nature at the center of our existence, and forests are the temple where the faithful go to look for a cure. Meditation in Buddhist temples is also almost always done in natural surroundings. Even in the city, meditation room windows usually give onto gardens full of trees. The walking meditation of Japanese Zen Buddhism known as *kinhin* is also preferably done in forests or gardens.

These traditions linking health and spiritual peace to nature weren't tested by science until the 1980s. But before we get into what Japanese scientists discovered when they researched the power forests have over health, which we'll go over in great detail in the next chapter, let's learn a bit about how poison in the right doses can make us stronger. To do so, we'll have to go back in history more than two thousand years.

The Universal Antidote of Mithridates VI the Great

The man who would be king of Pontus (Asia Minor) from 120 BCE until 63 BCE first had to get rid of his enemies, including his brother and his mother. He began suspecting them when his father, Mithridates V, was poisoned at a banquet, and his mother retained power because neither he nor his brother were old enough to govern. Suspecting that his mother had

----

7 We dedicated a chapter to this pioneering Japanese therapist in our first book, Ikigai: The Japanese Secret to a Long and Happy Life.

been the one to assassinate his father, Mithridates began to search for poison antidotes, and went to live in the woods far from his family. In order to immunize himself against possible assassination attempts, Mithridates began experimenting by taking low doses of snake venom. He also sometimes used imprisoned delinquents to try and find out how much of a dose wasn't lethal. Little by little he developed a mixture of vegetable and animal substances he called a "universal antidote," but which would historically become known as "mithridate." He discovered that taking small doses of this antidote gave him immunity to many poisons. The ingredients were listed and explained in one of the most important medical books of antiquity: *De Medicina*, by Aulus Cornelius Celsus, in year 30 of the Common Era. We refer to this 1st century formula below, although we advise against experimenting with it like the man who came up with it did.

THE FORMULATION OF MITHRIDATES

"It contains: costmary, 1.66 grams; sweet flag, 20 grams; hypericum, 8 grams; natural gum, 8 grams; sagapenum, 8 grams; acacia juice, 8 grams; Illyrian iris, 8 grams; cardamom, 8 grams; anise, 12 grams; Gallic nard (*Valeriana italica*), 16 grams; gentian root and dried rose leaves, 16 grams of each; poppy tears and parsley, 17 grams each; casia, saxifrage, darnel and long pepper, 20.66 grams of each; storax (liquid-ambar resin), 21 grams; castoreum, frankincense, hypocistis juice, myrrh, opopanax, and malabathrum leaves, 24 grams; flower of round rush, turpentine resin, galbanum, and carrot seeds, 24.66 grams of each; nard, opobalsam, and shepherd's purse, 25 grams of each; rhubarb root, 28 grams; saffron, ginger, and cinnamon, 29 grams of each.

- The ingredients are then pounded and taken up in honey.
- Against poisoning, a piece the size of an almond is given in wine. In other affections an amount corresponding in size to an Egyptian bean is sufficient."

—*De Medicina*, by Aulus Cornelius Celsus

After years of being away from home, Mithridates VI returned to the palace and killed his mother and brother to become king of Pontus. Legend has it that he developed such an immunity to poison that when he was defeated by Pompey, Mithridates VI tried to commit suicide by ingesting a large dose of poison. It didn't work, so he had to ask his friend Bituitus to kill him by the sword.

Mithridates didn't understand science, but he understood intuitively that the same poison that killed could also immunize if taken in low doses. As Paracelsus said back in the Middle Ages: "the dose makes the poison." In the modern age, this same principle was used to develop modern vaccines.

The Healing Powers of Phytoncides

Phytoncides are natural poisons. They were discovered in 1928 by the Russian biologist Boris P. Tokin who was experimenting in his lab when he identified the substances plants release to protect themselves. The function of these volatile organic compounds that are expelled by members of the plant kingdom is to prevent rot when a plant is being attacked by fungi or bacteria, or is being devoured by insects or animals. Humans are exposed to phytoncides when we eat vegetables, for example, but we're resistant to them because the doses are always so small. In fact, garlic (which has been a remedy for many types of diseases since antiquity) contains a very powerful type of phytoncide known as allicin. Today it is a component in pills used to treat certain diseases. Then there are the spices used in abundance in Far Eastern cooking which have a high phytoncide content and are known for their purifying and antibacterial power.

Another example we're all familiar with is the onion. In fact, phytoncides are what makes us cry when we chop onions. Technically, these substances are poison but at the right dosage they're good for us because their hormesis[8] is like the one in the potion Mithridates created, according to legend, to develop immunity. Spices, garlic, onions and all kinds of vegetables are healthy because they have a hormetic effect that we can understand using this graph.

----

8 Beneficial effects of ingesting a substance that would be toxic at higher doses. Caffeine is usually given as an example in that small doses are healthy, but too much can be bad for us.

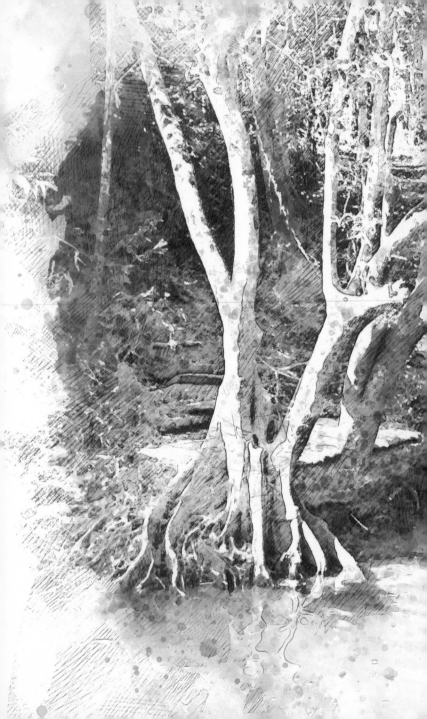

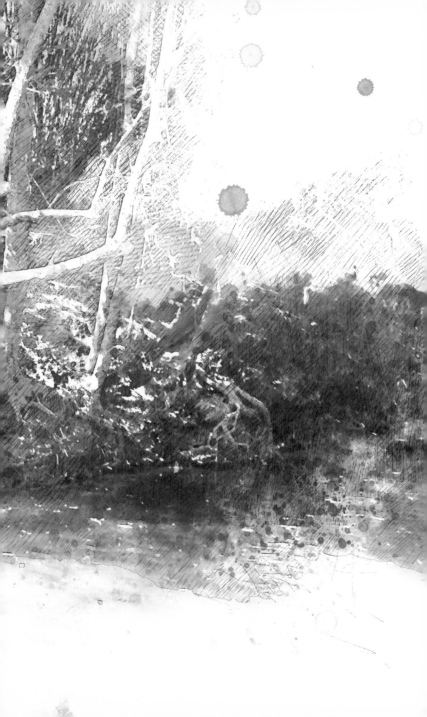

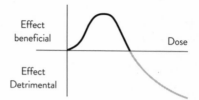

A substance or activity having hormetic effects follows a curve similar to the one on the graph. There's a point at which we're able to stimulate our system in a way that's beneficial, but if we go beyond it, the effects are detrimental.

The following table compares damage with hormetic effects to damage with detrimental, or harmful effects.

HORMETIC DAMAGE (beneficial at a certain dose)	DAMAGE DUE TO EXCESS
Being exposed to phytoncides in forests.	Taking these same compounds in concentrated form could be poisonous.
Physical exercise. (Sore muscles are due to having pushed our body, but we later benefit from hypertrophy, or muscle growth, which makes us stronger.)	Excessive exercise, many hours a day without taking precautions or resting properly. (Failure to rest means small growth tears are never repaired, so injury is more likely to occur.)
Alcohol. (At very low doses, it has hormetic effects.)	Too much alcohol is toxic, and has detrimental side effects.

HORMETIC DAMAGE	DAMAGE DUE TO EXCESS
(beneficial at a certain dose)	
Fasting or eating moderately. (Restricting calories kick starts autophagy in our cells, which reduces the probability of cancer cells proliferating.	Eating too much overloads the digestive system and accelerates the oxidation of cells. On the other end, too strict or continuous dieting damages the body and the nervous system, putting lives at risk due to disorders like anorexia.
Bathing in very cold or very hot water, up to a certain point, has been shown to provide excellent health benefits.	Hypothermia, if the temperature is too cold or exposure too lengthy. Burns, if the water is boiling.

However, not all substances have hormetic effects. Some can make us ill or even kill us with the smallest dose. Let's see some examples of agents that are only detrimental—agents that are toxic even at low doses.

- Breathing polluted urban gases.
- For those who are allergic, any exposure to allergens can be fatal (wasp stings, food allergies).
- Nicotine and other poisons from tobacco.

Phytoncides in Forests

In Part I we already pointed out that rates for depression and mental illness are higher in cities than in the countryside.

The question is, why are the benefits of being surrounded by nature so manifest? Scientific research in Japan began responding to this question in the 1980s, and found an explanation in the phytoncides discovered by the Russian biologist Boris P. Tokin half a century earlier.

In 1982, the Japanese Ministry of Agriculture, Forestry, and Fisheries initiated a national program to promote Japanese people's health based on the hypothesis that "bathing in the forest" was good for their health. This program was the first to propose using the word shinrin-yoku, a neologism in the Japanese language that combined the words *shinrin* (forest) and *yoku* (to bathe) in a single compound term.

Several research centers began to compare subjects who followed the national shinrin-yoku program and those who did not. Many studies were published, and though the results varied, nature was always favored. Scientists began to suspect that the trees' "poison"—phytoncides—favored hormonal changes that improve our health. Let's take a look at the conclusions and results from each of these studies to see how the hypotheses from the 1980s have recently been confirmed.

Reduction of Stress Hormones

The conclusion reached in one of the studies was that walking in the woods, or gazing at green space such as a garden, for example, reduces the concentration of cortisol in our saliva. Cortisol is a hormone associated with stress and anxiety.

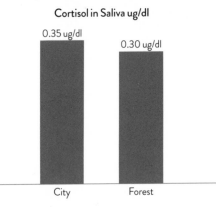

Cortisol in Saliva ug/dl

Lower Heart Rate

Another biomarker studied was heart rate, which is also lowered after walking in the forest, unlike what happens when we walk in the city. A lower heart rate was observed in subjects after they took a walk in green space, or simply sat down to contemplate nature.

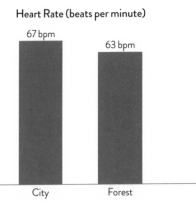

Heart Rate (beats per minute)

Lower Blood Pressure

Blood pressure was also measured in subjects showing lower heart rates, and it was found to be lower as well.

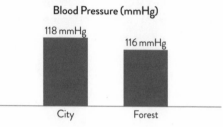

Heart Rate Variability (HRV)

Another biomarker measured was HRV (Heart Rate Variability), which the scientific community agrees is one of the key indicators for measuring our stress levels. This lets us know whether or not our autonomic nervous system[9] is functioning under stress. The greater our HRV, the better. In fact, scientists have shown that if our HRV is too low, the chances of dying in the next few years increase. One way to improve our HRV is to devote time to activities that are relaxing, and one of the most effective ways to do this is to meditate. Or just take a walk in the woods.

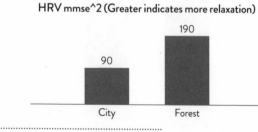

9 The autonomic nervous system is the part of the nervous system that controls all our involuntary actions.

Conclusions Regarding Stress Levels

If cortisol, heart rate and blood pressure, all of which are indicators of stress levels, are lowered at the same time that HRV (Heart Rate Variability) increases, the reliable conclusion is that all these biomarkers together demonstrate that walking in forests significantly reduces stress. It's not just a belief anymore; we have data to confirm it. Since 2017, smartwatches have begun to measure HRV, now that medical science gives vital importance to this key biomarker of stress.

Shinrin-yoku and NK Levels against Cancer

Everyone is afraid of cancer, but few are aware that within us we have a natural medicine that is very effective at destroying cancer cells. We're talking about NK cells. Short for Natural Killer, NK cells are a type of lymphocyte in our immune system, and they play an extremely important role in keeping us healthy. They can detect virus-infected cells as well as tumor cells. And not only do they detect them, they can eliminate them!

Imagine NK cells as part of a Pac Man game. Instead of moving across a screen eating up little dots, they move through our blood eliminating cancer cells. In several studies carried out in Japan by the Department of Hygiene and Public Health of Nippon Medical School, NK cell activity was analyzed in people exposed to natural surroundings, then compared with that of people who didn't leave the city. A group of subjects was sent on a two-night/three-day trip to the mountains in Nagano. Blood tests were done for each of them upon their return, and it was discovered that the number of NK cells had increased.

In order to be able to destroy cancer cells, our valuable NKs need to be loaded up with ammunition. In biological terms, NK cells use three proteins to work: GRN, perforin and GrA/B. When analyzing subjects' blood after the three days in Nagano, researchers found that the levels of these three proteins had also increased, meaning that the NK cells were working even better.

This graph shows the overall levels of NK cells, and the proteins needed for them to function well.

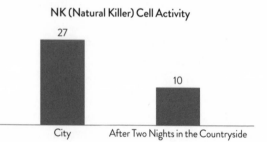

NK (Natural Killer) Cell Activity

The participants in the experiment not only had more NK cells after their stay in the forests of Nagano, but the cells were healthier and better equipped, ready to destroy cancer cells. In order to make sure these effects weren't just from walking or being relaxed on vacation, the same experiment was done with other subjects who spent three days as tourists in the city of Nagoya.

In this case, there was no difference in the activity of NK cells, their number or the expression of the three anticancer proteins: perforin, GRN and GrA/B. Another piece of good news this study uncovered was that, in the Nagano group, the effects at an NK cell level lasted up to seven days after the trip. This virtually provided proof that a weekend in the countryside has the power to improve our defenses against cancer for at least one week. This same scientific team conducted another experiment—just one day traveling to a wooded area outside Tokyo—and the effects were also similar. This indicated that a stroll through a wooded park on a Sunday has the power to protect us during the following week of life in the city.

The conclusion is clear: having a "forest bath" one day a week provides valuable protection against cancer, as well as other benefits. Of course, this kind of therapy doesn't mean patients should discontinue their treatment. In Japan, shinrin-yoku has been classified as preventive therapy, to help protect against illness, as well as reinforcement in recovery from operations or diseases.

Conclusions

The Japanese knew intuitively that exposure to nature was healthy for people. Later, in the 1980s, the first studies were conducted to show that patients who lived in green spaces improved sooner than those residing in cities, and this gave rise to the birth of the concept of shinrin-yoku. The hypothesis (unproven at the time) was that the phytoncides given off by trees and plants were the reason our health was improving, but no cause-effect relationship had been established. It wasn't until 2010 that conclusive studies were being published that showed a clear increase in the activity of NK cells, which are known for their ability to destroy cancer cells.

The question is: Why does NK cell activity increase when we walk in the woods? Are phytoncides really behind this increase, one that's so beneficial to our health? In addition to experiments with subjects in the countryside and in the city, others were also conducted in laboratories to definitively answer these questions. In one experiment, NK cells were used in vitro, or rather, NK cells were placed in Petri dishes together with phytoncides extracted from trees. What happened? When the phytoncides entered into contact with the NK cells, the latter were strengthened and they multiplied at a greater speed than those without contact with phytoncides. Science now had irrevocable proof that trees are a powerful medicine, something different traditions had known instinctively for millennia.

10 Major Health Benefits of *Shinrin-yoku* Proven by Science

We'll end the scientific part of this book by taking stock of what the numerous studies conducted in Japan have proven to date about the therapeutic power of forest bathing:

1. Strengthens the immune system, particularly the NK cells that directly fight tumor cells.

2. Contributes to reducing blood pressure and heart rate.

3. Reduces stress levels. Lowers levels of cortisol, a stress hormone.

4. Promotes serenity. Makes the nervous system less prone to "fight or flight" reactions.

5. Improves mood and a sense of well-being.

6. Increases ability to concentrate, even in children with ADHD.

7. Accelerates recovery following surgery.

8. Improves sleep.

9. Increases libido and sexual energy.

10. Improves visual health.[10]

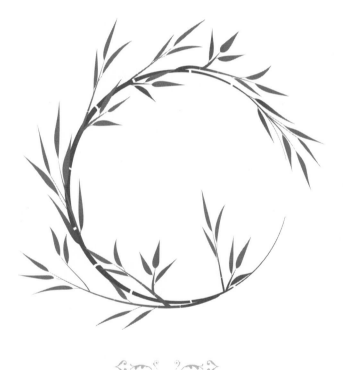

10 **Sources of Scientific Studies:**
All the graphs in this chapter show the average taken from all the participants in the study.
For readers with an understanding of statistics, the p-values are p<0.01.

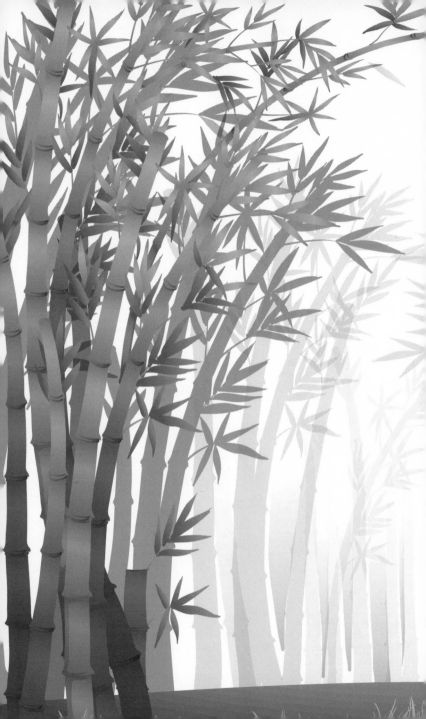

PART FOUR

The Philosophy
of *Shinrin-Yoku*

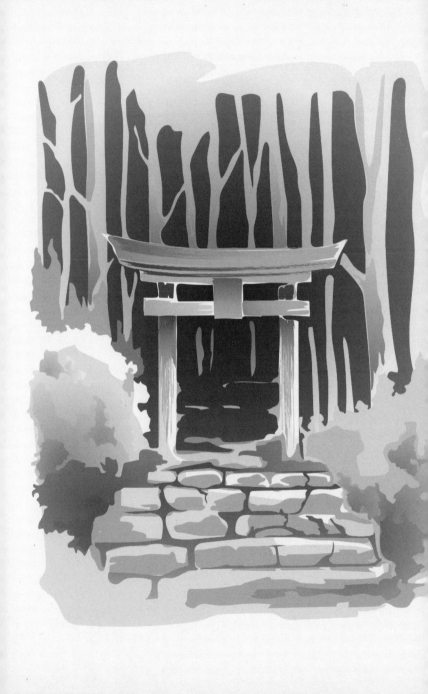

Shinto Spirits

Japan is one of the most technologically advanced countries in the world, yet as contradictory as it seems, tradition continues to carry a great deal of weight in all aspects of Japanese life. And it's remarkable that the two worlds rarely collide. The new blends harmoniously with the old: *geishas* using smart phones, school girls dressed in *yukatas*[11] and schoolboys in *jinbei*[12] in the summer, touch screen vending machines at the entrance to Buddhist temples, or professors walking around university campuses in wooden *getas*[13].

Respect for ancestors and tradition in general is ubiquitous in Japanese culture, and it's a value inherited from the Confucian religion originating in China. Another value embraced throughout the country is respect for nature, and this is inherent to Shinto, Japan's native religion. It can seem contradictory at first that a country having some of the largest megalopolises on the planet respects nature. But it turns out that Japan, despite being among the ten most developed countries in the world, has the largest area of forests and mountains, with 67% of its territory being forest cover.

Among the many themes addressed by Studio Ghibli productions, one is common to almost all of its films: nature. *Spirited Away* contains a very direct allegory: spirits contaminated by human trash have to be cleansed at the thermal baths. In *Princess Mononoke*, most of the action takes place in the woods where all kinds of creatures live, including *kodama*, tree spirits numbering in the hundreds, thousands and even

----

11 Traditional Japanese dress made up of a cotton kimono and belt
12 Two-piece garment, usually made of cotton, worn in the summer.
13 Traditional Japanese footwear reminiscent of wooden flip-flops.

millions. In Japan, belief is not in one all-powerful God; Shinto is an animistic religion in which spirits inhabit mountains, trees and rivers.

Ghibli is Shinto, nature, Japan.

A Call to the Spirits of Nature

When travelers who have just arrived in Japan enter a Shinto shrine, which is usually austere, even minimalist, they are often surprised by its bareness. Accustomed as Europeans are, in our case, to our impressive cathedrals, we might well think: is that all? But as visitors learn to value the simplicity of Shinto, they find that the beauty of its shrines begins to resonate in their hearts. The purpose of the Shinto shrine is not to overpower nature as something superior. It doesn't consist in demonstrating to the natural world what we humans are capable of, as many Western constructions attempt to do. On the contrary, Shinto shrines are intended to be integrated into nature in the most subtle way possible, for the purpose of calling to the spirits residing there to come communicate with us.

In Shinto, humans are part of nature, which we must honor as something superior while accepting that we are only part of its creation. Alan Watts makes a reflection that summarizes that vision well:

> "You didn't come into this world.
> You came out of it, like a wave from the ocean.
> You are not a stranger here."

Shinto, the ancient religion of Japan, is a system of local rituals and traditions that arose in these islands thousands of years ago, before the arrival of Buddhism, which was imported in the 6th century. Although both systems of beliefs are very different, there is a mysterious balance to the place they share in Japanese society. In numerical terms, Japan has about 80,000 Shinto shrines and about 55,000 Buddhist temples. Christianity is added in here to seal marriages. Typically, Japanese people celebrate birth following the Shinto ritual, marry in a Christian church, and end life with a Buddhist funeral. All these traditions are mysteriously interwoven.

There Is No One God

In its purest and most original form, Shinto consists in worshipping and admiring nature. Shinto has no sacred book; followers simply venerate mountains, forests and rivers. In antiquity, the Greeks also believed in a number of gods who lived on Mount Olympus, but this polytheism began disappearing in the West and Middle East with the arrival of Abrahamism. The seed of thought for these religions was the Platonic philosophy that portrays our reality as a mere copy of a perfect reality. Plato can partially be blamed for the idea of God as creator, superior to everything.

On the other hand, the dharmic religions that emerged in Asia, such as Hinduism or Buddhism, are more Aristotelian. According to Aristotelian physics, every object or being undergoes continuous change in order to become something "in the making." In the dharmic religions, everything in the universe is being necessarily transformed and changed. For example, one of the things that Buddhism teaches us is to accept change: death is inevitably going to come.

Potential, or possibility, exists within objects and beings; it's not something external that comes from a superior god. In this sense, Aristotle would be a Buddhist or Shintoist, for

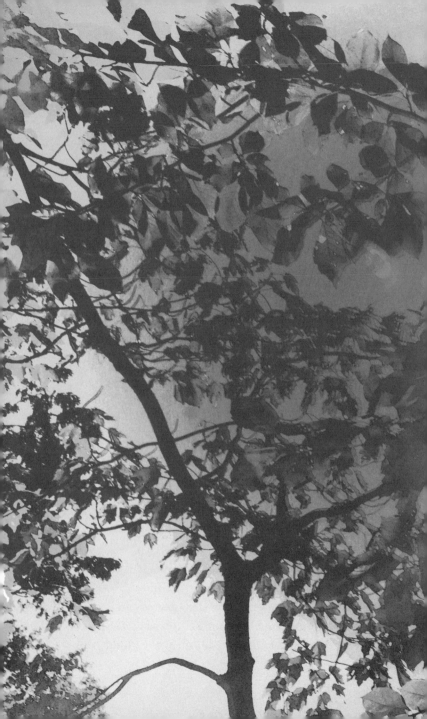

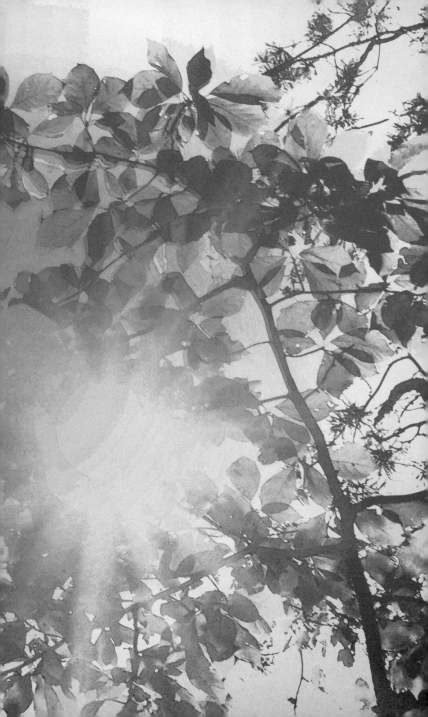

whom the spirit of every seed is to become a tree. Japanese Shinto is quite different from dharmic religions, but it shares this vision of continuous change and the idea that everything comes not from one God who created the world, but from gods numbering in the billions.

Kami: Spirits of the Forests, Rivers and Sea

According to Shinto tradition, there are billions of *kami*, spirits who inhabit the universe and have the power to appear in any element or force of nature. Kami move from here to there, and reside inside mountains, rivers, trees and plants. They can also appear in the form of storms, typhoons, earthquakes or volcanic eruptions. Kami can decide whether to do good or evil and, in this respect, parallels can be drawn with the gods on Mount Olympus. Worshipping kami in *Matsuri* (festivals) is one of the ways the Japanese pray for good fortune in the form of an abundant rice harvest, fertility, good luck in business, in studies, health and road safety.

SHINTO: WAY OF THE GODS

The Japanese characters for Shinto are 神道

The first character, 神, is *shin* when accompanied by another character, but is *kami* when written alone (this is very common in the Japanese language), and refers to the deities or spirits we mentioned earlier.

The second character, 道, is *to* and means "the way." The combination of both characters can be translated as "the way of the gods."

This second character, which can also be *do*, is used at the end of many Japanese arts, such as *chado* (the way of tea), *judo* (the way of flexibility) or *kendo* (the way of the sword). The way is metaphoric, in the sense that by practicing things we become better human beings.

The element we use to follow "the way" can be diverse. We might turn to *kami* within Shinto practice, delve into tea by means of a tea ceremony, or learn a martial art. The important thing in all these "ways" is to maintain discipline.

The way, 道, is the common thread connecting martial arts, Shinto, and all arts in general in Japan.

The Simple Origins of Shinto Shrines

The earliest version of a Shinto shrine consisted in placing a large rock or driving a tree branch into the ground at the edge of a forest. Soon rituals were carried out around the branch or rock to get kami to come out of the woods. The purpose was to attract good kami and get them to inhabit the branch or rock, and so bring in a good harvest, frighten off dangerous animals like wild boars or bears, make the women fertile, or just bring good luck to the village.

Little by little, the lowly rock or stick driven into the ground evolved to become four sticks held together with rope. The idea was the same: to create a space cordoned off by the four lines of rope, where kami could live and in this way benefit the people. This type of shrine still can be seen in many places in Japan.

Over time, these primitive structures made to attract kami evolved and turned into the Shinto shrines that are now all over the cities as well as the forests of Japan. Entrance to the sacred enclosure is marked by *torii*, simple gates made of wooden posts with one or two crossbeams at the top.

After passing the torii, visitors find themselves on sacred ground. In the enclosure defined by the gates, the main structures are the *honden* hall and the *haiden* hall. What's the difference between them? The honden are solely for kami, whereas the haiden can be visited by people. From the haiden, you can usually see the inside of the honden where, apparently, there is often nothing to see. The empty space is very reminiscent of the primitive four-pole-and-rope structures. Can there be anything more minimalist than empty space?

The honden is a building designed for nature's kami to inhabit, whereas the haiden lets us mortals approach the kami to ask them for good fortune. The purpose of a Shinto shrine is to offer the gods sanctuary so they won't abandon us, whereas the purpose of Western architecture is often to make an impression. In secular Japanese architecture, on the other hand, the facades of houses and buildings are minimalist in a way that doesn't stand out. This contrasts with Western architecture, as descended from Roman and Greek traditions where the main focus was on the temple facade.

SHINTO	MONOTHEISTIC RELIGIONS
Millions of *kami* with specific powers.	One all-powerful God.
Various superstitions and rites.	Fixed beliefs.

SHINTO	MONOTHEISTIC RELIGIONS
Wishes are made.	Sins are confessed.
There are no rules, just rituals that change with the times and the occasion.	Rules are established.
Integration of human beings in nature, in order to get *kami* to leave the forest and go to the shrine.	Temples and cathedrals that show the power of gods over what is human or natural.
Purpose: to coexist with nature as harmoniously as possible.	Purpose: salvation and eternal life.

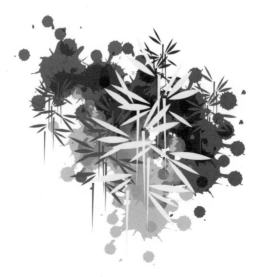

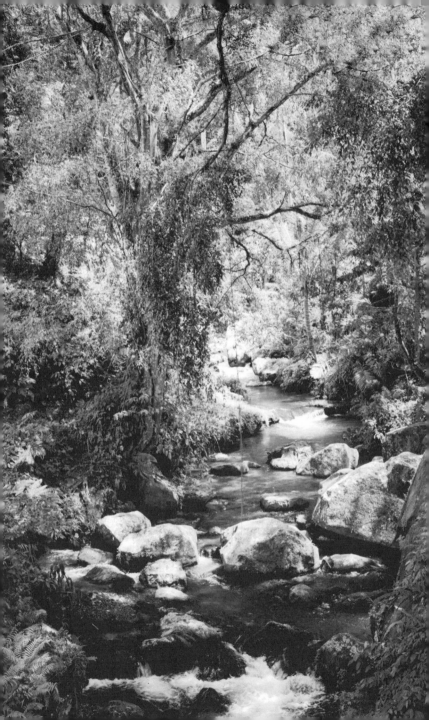

Yugen

In keeping with Shinto, many Japanese arts are intimately linked with nature. *Ikebana*, bonsai, traditional architecture (always working with wood and organic forms) and literature are closely related to artists' admiration for the natural world. In this chapter, we'll see how traditional poetry has always found sources of inspiration in the depths of the forests.

The Experience of Yugen 幽玄

The first character, 幽, means "deep, remote darkness"; the second character, 玄, means "mysterious or hidden." When put together, the two characters of this Japanese aesthetic might be translated as "the mysterious moments in which, while observing the universe, our feelings reach the depths of our innermost, hidden core." This is what people walking in the thick of the forest feel when the sun just barely filters through the leaves on the trees. Yet this aesthetic sensation isn't exclusive to contemplating nature. When we're enjoying art, for example, or listening to a delicate, melancholic piano piece, we can feel *yugen* deep inside us.

So, what exactly is yugen? It's what we experience when we gaze at a starry sky at night, when we suddenly lose our individuality the moment we realize we're part of something bigger than ourselves. It's a feeling that nature provokes in us: the moment we understand we aren't separate from the universe, that we are the universe. This deep, mysterious sense of the beauty of the cosmos is shared by everyone, but we can also cultivate it so we can summon those moments at will.

Evoking *Yugen*

Yugen can be felt not just in the depths of the forest or under a starry night sky. We can also awaken it within us through the arts. If we learn to appreciate painting, music and good literature, we'll be able to experience it and completely forget about our everyday problems. The Japanese say that poetry and *noh* theater are both excellent ways of evoking yugen.

Noh theater actors always perform wearing masks. This way, when the actors speak directly to the audience, each audience member feels like they are always the one being addressed. This is what creates the magic and mysterious feeling that they are also a part of the play's universe.

The Art of *Waka*

The literal meaning of *waka* is "Japanese poem," and there are many different styles, but the most significant ones are short poems, *tanka*, and long poems, *choka*. *Tanka* is a much older poetic form than *haiku* (which is a brief composition of three verses having five, seven and five syllables, respectively), and it uses nature as its source of inspiration. Japanese poetry also evokes yugen, as we can see in this choka by Zeami Motokiyo:

> To watch the sun sink behind a flower clad hill.
> To wander on in a huge forest without thought of return.
> To stand upon the shore and gaze after a boat
> that disappears behind distant islands.
> To contemplate the flight of wild geese
> seen and lost among the clouds.
> And, subtle shadows of bamboo on bamboo.

Shinrin-yoku and Yugen

In this poem, we see how nature has the power to awaken yugen in us, even if only by reading what a 14th-century poet felt. Sensitive-hearted people can feel yugen in the arts or, more directly, by practicing shinrin-yoku. When taking a walk in a field or a garden, we're hit with yugen in those moments of calm when we stop to unhurriedly contemplate the scenery around us. Standing before the beauty and immensity of natural surroundings, we feel we are merging with the mystery of creation.

Yugen exists at dawn and at dusk, as well as when we contemplate the raindrops making a puddle or the petals falling from the *sakura*, or cherry blossoms. When looking at the night sky, all you need in order to summon this feeling is to breathe deeply and close your eyes a moment. Imagine you're a traveler in a giant spaceship that is planet Earth. Visualize how our world crosses the stars. Open your eyes again and feel the yugen from the starry sky in all its splendor. We are cosmic travelers.

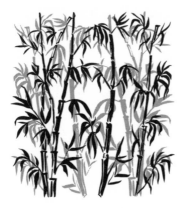

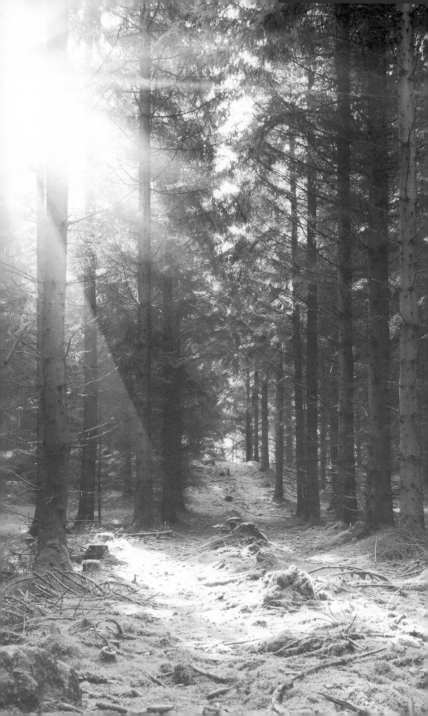

Komorebi

There is a Japanese word that is applied to the patterns of light and shade at play in the forest: *komorebi*. The Japanese appreciate the beauty in the chiaroscuro that varies depending on the types of trees, the wind and humidity, and the seasons. Komorebi encompasses all the effects of light and shade that nature can generate, whether it be the brightness of sun on leaves, the mysterious curtain that forms when there is fog, the thick humidity after it rains and the sun suddenly comes out, or the way the shadows of the leaves move on the forest floor.

ETYMOLOGY OF *KOMOREBI* 木漏れ日

木 =tree　漏れ =what sneaks through　日 =sunlight

The Japanese obsession with komorebi is apparent in many of the forest scenes in the film *Rashomon* by Akira Kurosawa, where illumination of the actors is based on areas of light and shade. This forest komorebi is also present in the Zelda videogame series with a level of detail that is very close to reality. Komorebi defines the dance between light and shade, a subject Tanizaki delved into in his small, classic essay, *In Praise of Shadows*. This untranslatable term is used for the patterns of light and shade generated by nature. When walking in the forest, knowledge of this concept will help us appreciate the beauty of the patterns made when the sun filters through the leaves of the trees. Komorebi is a work of abstract art created by nature.

Marion Milner's Revelation

A year after the publication of Tanizaki's *In Praise of Shadows*, the British psychoanalyst Marion Milner published *A Life of One's Own*. In this journal, written over seven years, the author wondered what made her happy and what she really wanted in life. She found the answer to these questions thanks to komorebi during a walk in the countryside. Milner lived right by a forest, and she walked there often. In one entry in her journal, she describes an occasion when the play of light and shade hypnotized her in such a way as to make her feel she was surrendering to the beauty of nature.

> One evening I saw that the half-opened leaves of trees by the dusty roadside, sycamores perhaps, made a pattern against the pale sky, like tracery of old iron-work gates or the decorations on ancient manuscripts. I had an aching desire to possess the pattern, somehow to make it mine—perhaps drawing would capture it.

After this revealing walk in the forest, Milner explains how the vision of komorebi brought about a change in the way she dealt with her vital worries, an invitation to feel more:

> If just looking could be so satisfying, why was I always striving to have things or to get things done? Certainly I had never suspected that the key to my private reality might lie in so apparently simple a skill as the ability to let the senses roam unfettered by purposes. I began to wonder whether eyes and ears might not have a wisdom of their own.

Being attentive to subtle, changeable designs, like the abstract imagery komorebi affords us, can trigger all sorts of ideas like the ones that possessed this observer who found her own therapist in the forest. Instead of walking around distractedly, or taking photos willy nilly, focusing our senses on this dance of chiaroscuro is an excellent way to meditate, and an invitation to enter into the subtle mysteries of the natural world.

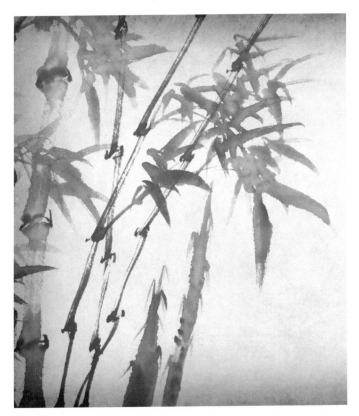

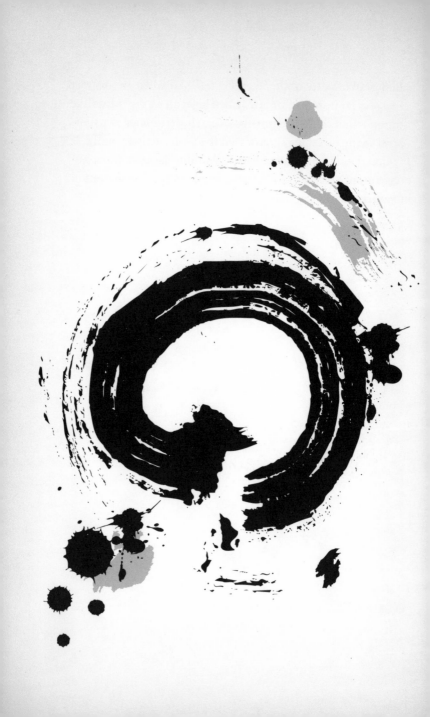

Wabi-sabi 侘寂

Aconcept unique to Japanese culture is *wabi-sabi*. Translated as "the beauty of imperfection," though there is much more to it than that, it was inspired by observations in nature. As the Catalan architect Antoni Gaudí said, there are no straight lines in nature, quite the opposite: it's full of asymmetry. Nothing is permanent either, as Buddha observed. Yesterday's green leaf is dry today, or may even have fallen off the tree. All this is encompassed by the philosophy of wabi-sabi, the aesthetic pillar of the Japanese people, and can be summarized in these three principles:

1. **Beauty is imperfect.** This is why an irregularly-shaped cup whose surface is rough or even cracked is much more highly valued than an impeccable, symmetrical piece of porcelain.

2. **Beauty is incomplete.** In nature nothing is finished, everything is under constant construction, just like the human spirit. Those who believe they have completed their training are, without doubt, the most ignorant. This is why master calligraphers use one brushstroke to draw open-ended *enso* circles. It's more beautiful when it's unfinished, just like life.

3. **Beauty is ephemeral.** Everything in nature is born and dies. Herein lies the drama, but also the beauty. If something were to last forever, we wouldn't value it. The dangling leaf, on the verge of falling from the tree, is an image full

of poetry because it embodies the essence of life: we only love what we might lose.

Fading Beauty

From a etymological point of view, wabi-sabi (*) is formed by two words that even separately are difficult to translate. The 12th-century poet Kamo no Chomei, author of well-known waka, defined the first term:

> Wabi is like the feeling of the evening sky in autumn, somber of color, hushed of all sound. Somehow, as if for reasons one should be able to call to mind, tears begin to flow un-controllably.

Makoto Ueda, professor emeritus of Japanese literature at Stanford University, completes the meaning of these two connected terms in this hazy, poetic way.

> *Wabi* originally meant "sadness of poverty." But gradually it came to mean an attitude toward life, with which one tried to resign himself to straitened living and to find peace and serenity of mind even under such circumstances. *Sabi*, pri-marily an aesthetic concept, is closely associated with *wabi*, a philosophical idea.

Wabi-sabi is, therefore, the aesthetics of sadness or poverty that gives us serenity of mind. Simply put: the beauty of im-perfection. Many people feel more peace of mind working at a table amid a bit of clutter than at a perfectly neat desk where every move we make threatens the very order of the universe. Just the way old shoes are more comfortable than the new pair that end up giving us blisters, things that are imperfect, incomplete and ephemeral give us the placidness that nature inspires.

Andrew Juniper summarizes:

> *Wabi sabi* is an intuitive appreciation of a transient beauty in the physical world that reflects the irreversible flow of life in the spiritual world. It is an understated beauty that exists in the modest, rustic, imperfect, or even decayed, an aesthetic sensibility that finds a melancholic beauty on the impermanence of things.

Tsurezuregusa: Essays in Idleness

Inspired by nature, this aesthetic concept can be a focus for reflection when we practice shinrin-yoku. The realization that no two walks can be exactly the same, that our feet will never step on the same bit of earth again, makes the experience unique and unrepeatable. If you aren't paying attention to the wonders of the forest here and now, you'll never be able to enjoy them.

This feeling of being temporary clashes with the human longing to make things permanent, what Buddha saw as the source of our suffering. This was something Yoshida Kenkó wrote about in the 14th century in his *Tsurezuregusa* (Essays in Idleness). The author, like Thoreau, lived in a cabin in the middle of the woods, though he wrote his thoughts on pieces of paper that he pasted to the walls of his cottage. When Yoshida died, a good friend of his carefully removed these scraps of paper, 243 in all, and collected them in what would become a classic in Japanese literature. Among other things, it discusses how ephemera make us happy:

If man were never to fade away... but lingered on forever in the world, how things would lose their power to move us. The most precious thing in life is its uncertainty. Consider living creatures—none lives so long as man. The May fly waits not for the evening, the summer cicada knows neither spring nor autumn. What a wonderfully unhurried feeling it is to live even a single year in perfect serenity. If that is not enough for you, you might live a thousand years and still feel it was but a single night's dream.

The Wisdom of a Japanese Grandmother

In *Living Wabi Sabi: The True Beauty of Your Life*, the American author Taro Gold details the lessons he learned from his Japanese grandmother on how to live under the serene beauty of imperfection.

People often fantasize that lasting joy will come to them as a result of perfection....Most people dream of the perfect mate, the perfect job, the perfect home and so on. But to wish for perfection is to deny reality. It actually invites the opposite of what we seek. Perfection exists only in the imagination. As long as we equate joy with perfection, even in a small way, we will never know contentment.

The ancient Wabi Sabi masters understood this well... They knew that happiness does not mean "absence of problems." There has never been, nor will there ever be, a life free from problems. Since there is no such thing as a perfect life, Wabi Sabi teaches us a way of looking at life that accepts imperfections, makes peace with the difficulties and mishaps, and strives to use them for our ultimate enrichment.

Abandoning our useless need for control and going into the woods can mark the difference between the quest for perfectionism, which makes us suffer, and the freedom to let life unfold in its own way beneath our feet. In this sense, there is no particular destination for wabi-sabi walking. It's better to improvise walks and be surprised along the way, to let ourselves be guided by intuition and a moment's inspiration. With this spirit of relaxed improvisation, a long, imperfect walk can end up being a most perfect and happy experience.

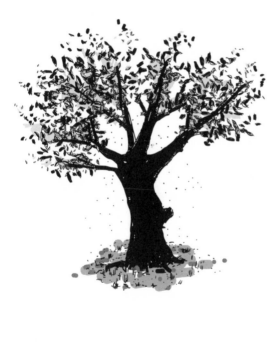

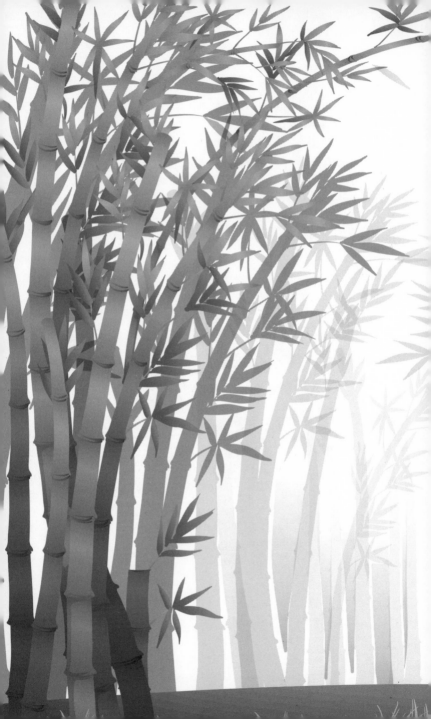

PART FIVE

The Practice of *Shinrin-Yoku*

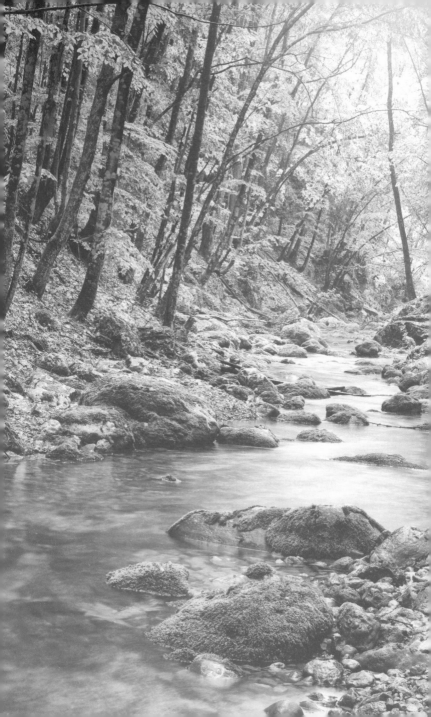

Return to the Forest

"The clearest way into the Universe is through a forest wilderness," said John Muir. Born in Scotland in 1838, Muir later emigrated to the United States and was so impressed by its wilderness that he became one of the first and most important activists in nature conservation. His influence was so great that these days Muir is known in the United States as the "father of National Parks," and several mountains and peaks in different states bear his name.

As it happens, John Muir was a key figure in making Yosemite a national park. The conservation area in California, familiar to us these days thanks to Apple computer screen wallpaper and Ansel Adams photographs, was declared a national park in 1890. Although the naturalist was instrumental in achieving this goal, regulations at the time weren't very strict, and the area continued to be exploited by logging companies, in addition to being artificially remodeled by builders who worked for the state.

The final step in convincing the government that this lack of respect for nature needed to end completely (and not just partially) was an incident in the early 20th century when Muir accompanied President Theodore Roosevelt to Yosemite. They were on a three-day wilderness trip when the two of them left the presidential delegation behind and headed into the deep woods. They camped at one of the most beautiful sites in the park, Glacier Point, where they talked under the stars well into the night. In the morning they woke to fresh snow falling softly on the forest around them. The president was so impressed with the adventure that he spent the following years making stricter regulations to protect not just Yosemite, but other natural US treasures as well.

Near the end of his life, Theodore Roosevelt declared that that he had never been able to forget that night with John Muir in the heart of Yosemite. The tenacious naturalist took the first steps in putting the brakes on the predatory effects of the Industrial Revolution in the 19th century. Following his lead, many other countries adopted measures to protect natural spaces, and today it's common practice in most developed countries.

INSPIRING QUOTES FROM JOHN MUIR

In addition to fighting to protect forests, John Muir was an acclaimed writer. Nature is always present in his texts, and in the United States he continues to be a huge source of inspiration. Written more than a century ago, his words are an invitation to indulge in *shinrin-yoku*:

"Keep close to Nature's heart... and break clear away, once in awhile, and climb a mountain or spend a week in the woods. Wash your spirit clean."

"In every walk with nature one receives far more than he seeks."

"Rocks and waters, etc., are words of God, and so are men. We all flow from one fountain Soul. All are expressions of one Love.."

"In the eternal youth of Nature you may renew your own. You see the nature in silence, nothing will do damage to you."

"Going to the woods is going home."

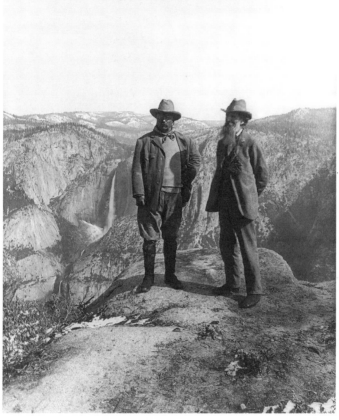

John Muir acting as guide for President Theodore Roosevelt in Yosemite (1906)

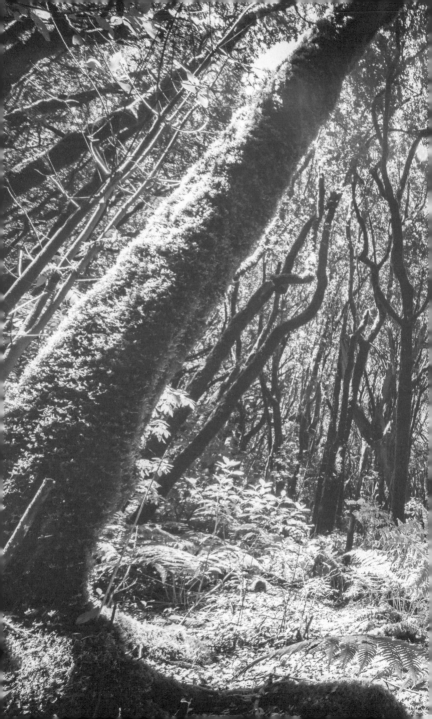

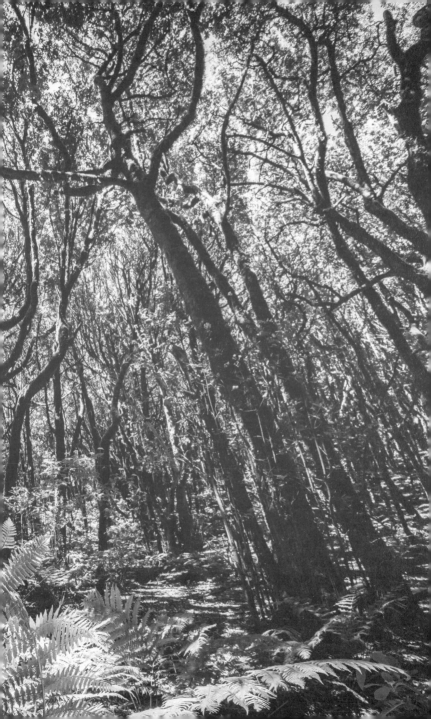

Return of the Forests

In Spain, the first natural space to be declared a national park was Picos de Europa, in 1916, a territory that extends across the provinces of Asturias, Leon and Cantabria. This was followed by Ordesa and Monte Perdido in Huesca, and Teide in Tenerife. These were the first three, but today Spain has fifteen national parks.

In Japan there are thirty-four national parks, and one of the best known among travelers is Yakushima. An almost magical volcanic island, it's completely covered in mountains and trees, many of which are more than a thousand years old, and some, it is said, could be over seven thousand. Native sika deer and monkeys move with complete freedom around the island, unafraid of visiting tourists. This wilderness has inspired many Japanese artists; for example, the forests in the film *Princess Mononoke* are modeled on Yakushima.

Though we might think our polluted, overpopulated civilization is eating up the forests, data would suggest the opposite is true. Forest area in developed countries is growing. In the past two decades, forests in Italy and Greece have gone from covering 26% of the territory to 32%. In the case of Spain, the growth of forests is even more spectacular, showing an increase in forest area from 28% in 1990 to the current rate of 37%.

The two major reasons for this growth are thought to be:
- Conservation promoted by government agencies.
- Crop cultivation being abandoned in many areas, which means forests have been allowed to encroach on many areas that had once been agricultural.

This situation is the opposite in other places in the world. For example, millions of acres of forest are lost every year in the Amazon jungle. It's also a huge problem in Africa, where deserts are encroaching on green spaces. We've come a long way since John Muir took the first step in forest conservation, but we still have a long way to go.

From National Parks to *Shinrin-yoku*

Thanks to the work of nature advocates, people and governments have understood the importance of protecting forests in their purest state. As to the practice of shinrin-yoku, it's on its way to becoming established as something important as well.

In Japan, it has gotten to the point where there are now specific places (parks, gardens and wooded areas) that are specially designated for practicing shinrin-yoku, and people of all ages are being encouraged to visit them and reap the health benefits they offer.

Shinrin-yoku is an invitation to return to the forests. Several governmental agencies and non-profit organizations have set up more than one hundred official routes for practicing shinrin-yoku in Japan. The idea is to find spaces to be shared by humans and nature so that they intermingle in harmony. But let's look at the requirements generally met by official places in Japan for practicing shinrin-yoku:

- Abundance of all kinds of vegetation.
- Easy to walk without becoming strenuous. These routes are apt for children as well as for the elderly.
- Places where silence reigns, except for the sounds of nature.

The fundamental difference between these spaces and national parks or hiking routes would therefore be accessibility. Millions of Japanese people affected by stress, hypertension and anxiety from modern urban life turn to shinrin-yoku at one of the hundred or so official areas designated by the Forest Agency of Japan.

A PERSONAL EXPERIENCE

"Hey, wanna go *shinrin-yoku*?" a coworker asked me years ago. Since I didn't know the word then, I thought he wanted to go out for sake or some kind of meal.

"It's a type of preventive medicine and it's covered by our company's insurance," he went on as I raised my eyebrows. "It involves taking a walk in a forest on the outskirts of Tokyo."

That weekend, the whole team went to a forest deemed suitable for practicing *shinrin-yoku* by our health insurance. It was a wonderful day spent walking in nature. Ever since, we go once a year and our health insurance pays for transportation to the start of the route.   —Héctor

Once a Week

Although some Japanese companies provide annual employee outings, as we saw in Part III, the Science of Shinrin-yoku, a weekly stroll in greenery would be ideal for us to begin to feel the positive effects of this therapy on our health.

Spain now has its first official shinrin-yoku site, in the town of Sant Hilari Sacalm, Girona. The town hall there has teamed up with the Sèlvans Association to begin organizing three-hour therapeutic routes led by a guide. In Catalonia, this is the start of a network of old-growth forests (*Red de Bosques Maduros*) chosen for their natural richness and biodiversity to provide the psychological and physiological benefits of this practice.

Nevertheless, shinrin-yoku is within everyone's reach. Even if there is no designated route nearby, all anyone has to do is take a walk in the nearest green space. Look for a path surrounded by nature and silence. Find a place to reconnect with nature and just start walking and breathing at a leisurely pace. The next chapter will show us how to make the most of its benefits.

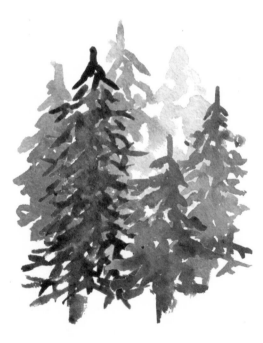

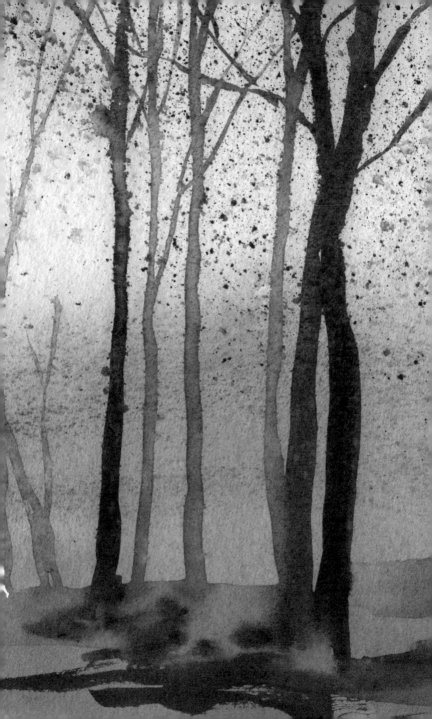

The 5 Steps of *Shinrin-yoku*

J ust taking a walk in a green space is enough to take in most of the benefits we saw in Part III. In the next chapter, a practical one, we'll explain how to take the greatest advantage of this "forest bathing."

Before getting to the five steps, it's important to prepare ourselves mentally to enjoy shinrin-yoku. In order to do so, we need to leave behind our daily worries, commitments and pending obligations—anything that will distract us from enjoying the here and now of the woods. Like the Celtic heroes who entered the sacred forest, or the native teen entering the forest as a rite of passage, we will interrupt our daily life for a few hours and give ourselves over completely to the experience.

These are the five steps that will help you fully enjoy shinrin-yoku:

1. **Give Yourself Up to the Experience, Here and Now**
    - For forest bathing to be effective, you need to give up multitasking. Set your phone to airplane mode and put it away, somewhere out of reach.
    - Be aware of each step, the temperature, the breeze, the play of light. The purpose of shinrin-yoku is for you to be absolutely present in the forest, evading nothing.
    - Just as having a cup of tea in a bar while discussing sports or politics is not the same as sitting on a tatami looking onto a forest and talking about the sound of rain, intention is essential to your walk. Walk in silence or, if accompanied, avoid chatting about worldly or stressful topics.

2. Have a Route in Mind, but Leave Room to Improvise

- Don't be in a hurry or worried about reaching a certain point in an itinerary. All your attention should be on walking placidly, breathing and stopping wherever your imagination dictates.
- Give yourself permission to sit on a rock or a fallen tree trunk if you feel fatigued. Enjoy the universe of sounds that fill the forest: birds, cicadas, the leaves rustling in the wind... Breathe in the fresh, revitalizing aromas of the forest.
- Go another way if you come upon a more attractive path. Hand the compass over to your feet so they can follow a moment's inspiration.
- Stop to admire the scenery, especially at dusk or dawn.

3. Take Slow, Deep Breaths

- In addition to walking at a leisurely pace, letting yourself be enveloped by nature and clearing your mind, the purpose of shinrin-yoku is to breathe. Do this in a relaxed, deep way, whether you're walking, standing still, sitting or lying under the shelter of a tree.
- When you take slow breaths, mobilizing your belly, lungs and collarbones, visualize as they rise how the beneficial phytoncides are absorbed deep inside you. Each time you inhale, take in the rush of nature's healing.
- Feel yourself being flooded in greenery, bathe your body and your mind in this sensation.

4. Let Your Mental Clouds Pass By

- Accustomed as you are to the constant distractions clouding your mind, troubling thoughts may come to you in the midst of shinrin-yoku. Don't panic, that's normal.

- Take deep breaths and picture these worries as clouds in the sky of your mind. They float from one side to the other until the wind blows them away. Label them as "thoughts" and let them pass by, without rejecting or retaining them, without analyzing or judging them. They're just thoughts that come and go like little clouds that get lost in the distance, finally allowing you to feel the present.
- If you feel stressed by the tensions of the week, take a break in your walk to do some stretching, *tai chi* or *qigong* positions[14], right there in the forest.

5. Feel Yourself as Part of Everything

- Anchored in the here and now, absolutely present, you will begin to feel integrated in the forest, nature, the whole universal.
- Experience yugen, the magic of being at one with the plants and animals around you, with all human beings, with this beautiful planet warmed by a distant star.
- Accept that you are an important part of the universe, not something separate from it. You are the universe and the universe is you. Let your ego dissolve into the surroundings until you become one with nature. Going back to Alan Watts: "You are a function of what the whole universe is doing in the same way that a wave is a function of what the whole ocean is doing."

----

14 Chapter VIII of our book, *Ikigai: The Japanese Secret to a Long and Happy Life*, has step-by-step illustrations for doing these easy exercises.

WHAT TO DO DURING *SHINRIN-YOKU*

Be aware and focused only on the experience.

Empty your mind.

Forget about time and pressing needs.

Walk leisurely, stop when you need to, breathe.

Talk about what you observe in nature.

Look for silent spaces.

Anchor yourself in the present.

Forget about having to get home.

WHAT NOT TO DO DURING *SHINRIN-YOKU*

Get distracted by your smart-phone (turn it off or set it to air-plane mode).

Go over problems, commitments or worries.

Watch the clock or be in a hurry to complete the route.

Make a sport of the long walk.

Talk about politics, sports or stressful news.

Spend the whole time chatting.

Brood over the past or the future.

Spend the whole time thinking about having to get home and what has to be done when you get there.

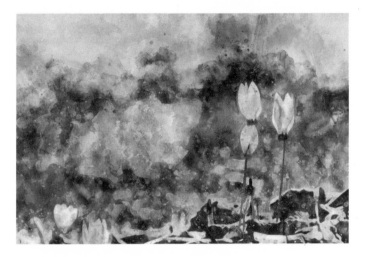

Take the Spirit of the Forest Home

After experiencing shinrin-yoku, it's important to make a gradual return to urban life, making sure we feel, in our calmer mind and body, all the benefits gained from our walk. For days after our "forest bath" we'll have recourse to a valuable reserve of calm for whenever we feel stressed. During the next week, if we again feel anxiety praying on us, we can just close our eyes, breathe deep and visualize some of the places we visited on our route. Soon we'll remember what we felt on our walk in nature, and the serenity found in the forest will return.

In the next chapter, we'll dig a little deeper into these five basic steps for practicing shinrin-yoku, and we'll learn techniques for meditating in the forest.

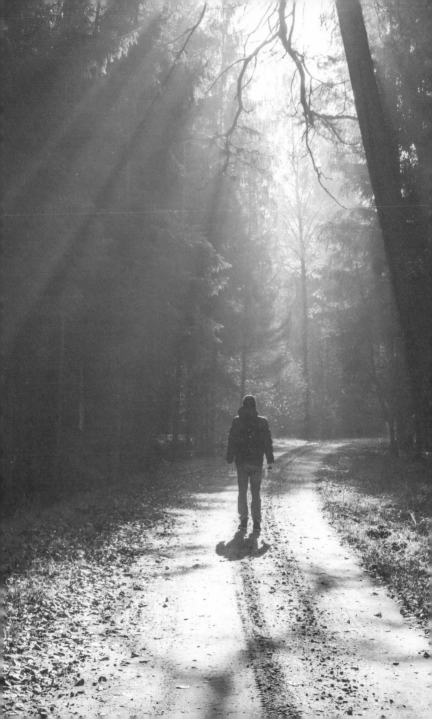

Mindfulness in the Outdoors

Even before the physician Jon Kabat-Zinn popularized the term "mindfulness" and designed the first courses for the Western world, the monk Thich Nhat Hanh began teaching techniques for meditating and being present anywhere. In the midst of nature as well. This Vietnamese Zen Master, author of more than a hundred books and nominated several times for the Nobel Peace Prize, says that mindfulness isn't something to be confined to a classroom or meditation room. It can radiate into every aspect of our lives, even when we go for a walk outdoors.

WALKING MEDITATION IN THE FOREST

"Wherever we walk, we can practice meditation. This means that we know that we are walking. We walk just for walking. We walk with freedom and solidity, no longer in a hurry. We are present with each step. And when we wish to talk we stop our movement and give our full attention to the other person, to our words and to listening.

Walking in this way should not be a privilege. We should be able to do it in every moment. Look around and see how vast life is, the trees, the white clouds, the limitless sky. Listen to the birds. Feel the fresh breeze. Life is all around and we are alive and healthy and capable of walking in peace.

Let us walk as a free person and feel our steps get lighter. Let us enjoy every step we make. Each step is nourishing and healing. As we walk, imprint our gratitude and our love on the earth.

—Thich Nhat Hanh

In fact, one of the purposes of meditation is to extend full awareness to all acts in our daily lives. Besides meditating while sitting and meditating while walking as the Vietnamese master proposes, Zen monks try to incorporate the same level of attention into all the day's activities, from sweeping the floor to washing a potato. With this mindfulness, life becomes a constant flow whereby subject and action are the same thing. Almost the equivalent of a home version of yugen.

Haptic Perception

If we analyze our way of living a bit, we'll see that in our perception of the world certain senses take precedence over others. So today's society has become eminently audio-visual, and this means that two senses have eclipsed the other three. From earliest childhood, kids grow up connected to videogames that involve only sight and sound, just like the films and series that fill the time of both children and adults. The other three senses—taste, touch and smell—are clearly underutilized. These are classified under haptic perception, which refers to all the sensations we experience in addition to sight and hearing.

Taste would be the third sense, in order of importance, for gourmets and anyone who likes good food, but the senses of smell and touch have been increasingly relegated. Unlike our counterparts in the animal kingdom, we have lost the ability to detect smells, even at close range. When it comes to touch, we use it less and less often; we barely use our hands at all to explore our surroundings. Shinrin-yoku provides an excellent opportunity to regain haptic perception, to once again perceive the world using all of our senses.

Meditate in Nature Using All Five Senses

This exercise can be practiced in the woods or an urban garden. What's important is that we be surrounded by greenery. We can do it lying down or sitting, even on a park bench. Bring something small to eat, like raisins or nuts, or even a bit of chocolate. After taking a few long, deep breaths, ask yourself these questions:

What do you see?
- Watch the branches as they move, the birds, fallen leaves, flying insects.
- Notice the play of light and shadow, *komorebi*.
- Look at old tree trunks, worn rocks, nature's *wabi-sabi*.
- Take in all the different colors and the contrasts between them.

What do you hear?
- Pay attention to the symphony of sounds around you.
- Try to separate and identify each of them, as if you were listening for the different instruments in an orchestra.

What do you smell?
- With your eyes half closed now, breathe deep and inhale the forest aromas all around you.
- Try to pick out the scent of flowers, fresh leaves, damp earth.

What can you touch?
- Reach your hands out and softly touch a plant, a rock, or even the ground.
- Explore rough bark, a cold, smooth stone, the fragile

stem of a plant.

- Feel the temperature in your body, the cool breeze, the caress of air going in and out of your nostrils.
- If you're standing up, take your shoes off and feel the texture of the soil, your weight on the ground. Take a few deliberate steps to really feel it.

What does it taste like?

- Bring the small bit of food you have to your mouth.
- First hold it between your lips, noticing the texture.
- Then put it on your tongue so your saliva can begin to break down its flavor.
- Finally bite and chew to squeeze all the juice out.

Field notes

Spaniards born in the late 60s or earlier will remember a collection of "field notes" by the great naturalist Félix Rodriguez de la Fuente. They were brown booklets full of drawings and sketches, observations on nature made with hand-written notes. To help us delve deeper into all five senses, it can be very useful to carry a small notebook and pen or pencil to note the following:

- What we perceived with each one of our senses.
- Sketches of the natural elements that interested us the most.

On the other hand, reading or writing haiku, which are almost always centered on nature, can really wake up our senses. In this regard, we'll very briefly recall the rules for writing haiku that we mention in our book *The Ikigai Journey*.

1. Haiku have three non-rhyming verses.

2. Their brevity should be such that they can be read aloud in one breath.

3. Preferably, they should include some reference to nature or the seasons of the year.

4. Haiku are always set in the present (though verbs can be omitted), never turning to the past or the future.

5. They should express a poet's observation or wonder.

6. One (or more) of the five senses should be present in the verses.

In order to illustrate this poetic art—a form that gathers the essence of nature in a single moment and place—we'll end this chapter with haiku from the great Matsuo Basho:

> The winter storm
> hid in the bamboo grove
> and quieted away.

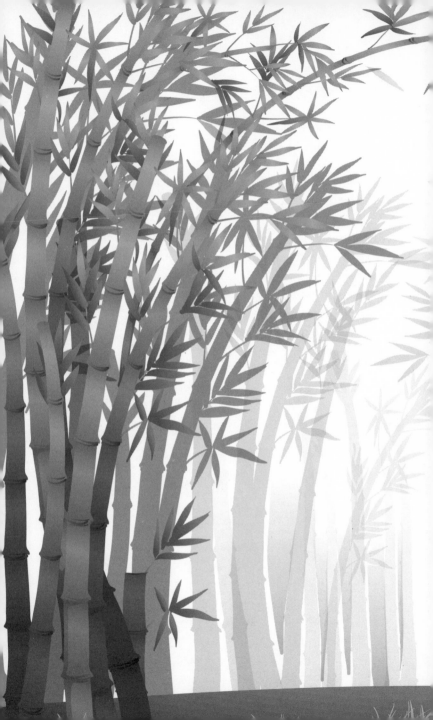

PART SIX

Shinrin-Yoku at Home

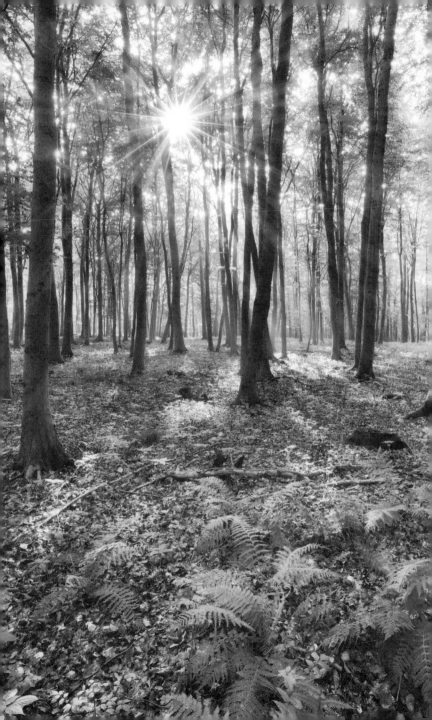

A Green Home

Practicing shinrin-yoku one day a week, or even more often if possible, can be supplemented by having a home that is literally as well as metaphorically green.

Green hues have proven to be relaxing for human beings, as well as favoring physical and psychological recovery. It's no coincidence that green is the "color of hope," because it subconsciously sends us back to our original habitat, where everything is reborn and renewed. This is why decorating a house with paintings and photographs centered on nature has a calming effect. In the same way, watching documentaries and films shot in large forests or jungles is a balm for the spirit, especially after a stressful day.

A WINDOW TO THE WOODS

If we can't get to nature as much as we would like due to our routines or where we live, we can absorb some of its serenity through television. There are thousands of excellent documentaries on the world's natural treasures, as well as specialized channels and fictional films where the forest is a main character.

The authors of this book have a favorite, which is *Dersu Uzala* (1975). The first film Japanese director Akira Kurosawa made abroad, and the only one he filmed in 70 mm., narrates the expeditions in the Siberian taiga of a group of Russian soldiers surveying the Ussuri river basin. There they meet Dersu Uzala, a kind-hearted nomadic hunter who acts as their guide and gives them important lessons on the secrets of nature and the human soul.

Healing Houseplants

We call them houseplants, but they could be called "personal plants," because they're so beneficial to our personal health and harmony. We mentioned one of their benefits at the beginning of this chapter: the color green, which has the power to calm us and help us rest. However, it's also clear that having plants in the home improves air quality, thanks to photosynthesis, which absorbs dioxide and releases necessary oxygen, thereby purifying the environment.

In her book *El Paraíso Es Su Casa* (Paradise Is Your Home), the Chinese-American author Diana Quan includes the following advantages to having houseplants: "They've been proven to remove toxins from the air. Although we can't see these so-called 'volatile organic compounds,' they're everywhere: carpets, trash bags, paintings, vinyl surfaces, synthetic fibers, cigarette smoke and even ink."

There are numerous studies on the benefits of houseplants, most of which point to the aforementioned calming effect of the color green. Others have shown that when there are plants in office environments, employees request fewer days off in a year, and their levels of concentration improve while stress levels decrease. But the most impressive results were obtained by NASA in several studies verifying that plants capture dust particles (many that are harmful to us, such as benzene molecules) and send them into the ground under their roots, where they become food for the same plants. This means that, besides eliminating CO_2, plants also eliminate all kinds of polluting particles from the air!

All plants have the ability to absorb harmful particles from the air, but according to results from NASA's study, one of the most powerful plants is *Sansevieria trifasciata*, commonly called mother-in-law's tongue or snake plant. It's particularly effective at eliminating benzene toxins, nitrogen oxide and trichloroethylene from the air. In Tokyo, this is one of the most common houseplants, seen as often in subway stations as in offices.

OTHER HEALING PLANTS

NASA researchers concluded that, in addition *to Sansevieria trifasciata*, the best plants for removing toxins from the air are:

- *Dracaena reflexa*, native to Mozambique.
- *Epipremnum aureum*, better known as golden pothos or devil's ivy.
- Chrysanthemum.
- *Spathiphyllum*, commonly known as spath or peace lilies.

Another fun fact about houseplants is that they absorb noise, which is why it's a good idea to keep plants near windows in the city. As we've seen, keeping a bit of the forest at home provides all sorts of benefits, and this is something ancient cultures have always known. In India, for example, basil has been used for thousands of years to clean houses and foster a sense of peace.

The ancient rules of *feng shui*, says Diana Quan, also value the power of houseplants to balance *chi* energy within the home, giving a boost to our emotional and physical well-being. According to this Chinese method: "Not all plants can be considered beneficial. This is the case with bonsais, because they symbolize an energy whose development was atrophied, and with dried flowers, because their *chi* is dead [...] All plants need to be well cared for, healthy and arranged in a harmoni-

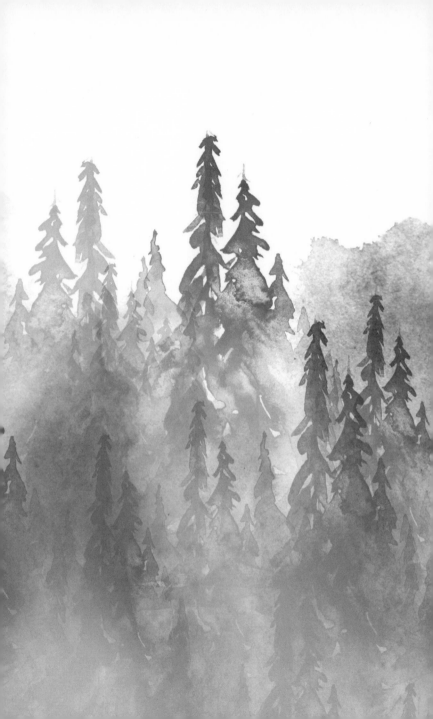

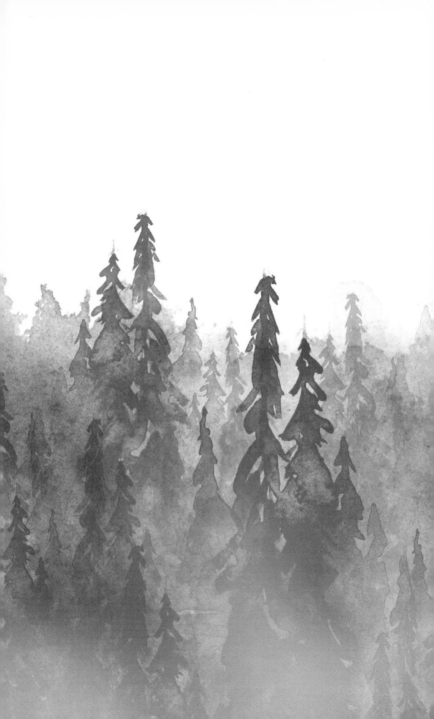

ous fashion. They shouldn't be left to grow any which way, or to wilt, as this transmits negative energy to the environment."[15]

Essences and Phytoncides

In the chapter on science, we saw that one of the keys to the valuable effects of shinrin-yoku are phytoncides. Can we get the same effect without leaving the house? Not exactly, but we can take advantage of part of its properties with the help of essential oils.

All we need to get started in aromatherapy is to buy a diffuser and good quality oils. A good place to put one, for example, is next to the computer where we work. Besides providing phytoncides, different essential oils have the ability to influence our mood. After a diffuser has been on for a half an hour, particles stay in the air for three or four hours.

Any essential oil has effects similar to those we saw in the chapter on science, but the most effective ones seem to be oils that have been extracted directly from trees because they have a greater concentration of phytoncides. Let's look at a few that have proven to be more effective.

I. **Cypress Oil.** In a study conducted in Japan, *hinoki* (Japanese cypress) essential oil was used to vaporize hotel rooms. This is the same oil that was used in Petri dish experiments to prove that they activated our highly-valued NK cells, which are fundamental in keeping cancer cells at bay. When conducting this new experiment on subjects who were staying in hotel rooms, having no contact with nature

---

15 Translator note: Translated into English from the Spanish.

but breathing air vaporized with cypress oil, an increase in health and NK cell activity was observed. All in all, there was a 20% increase in activity over another group of subjects at the same hotel who were in rooms without aromatherapy.

2. **Pine Oil.** In another study, *sugi* essential oil (Japanese pine) was used with subjects who spent several days in rooms with aromatherapy. Subsequent medical checkups showed a reduction in blood pressure and stress.

3. **Cedar Oil.** Lastly, another test showed that a group using a diffuser with cedar essential oils on a daily basis achieved a significant reduction in blood pressure compared to another group that wasn't exposed to aromatherapy.

Other essential oils with a significant phytoncide content are eucalyptus, any conifer oil, and oils from citrus trees. There are some essential oils that have a lower concentration of phytoncides, but they have other health benefits. An important thing to remember is to be aware of their properties before using them.

Finally, we'll see an example of how these six essential oils work.

RELAXATION
(to use at night, before bed)

Rose
Lavender
Chamomile

ACTIVATION
(to use in the morning)

Mint
Ginger
Orange

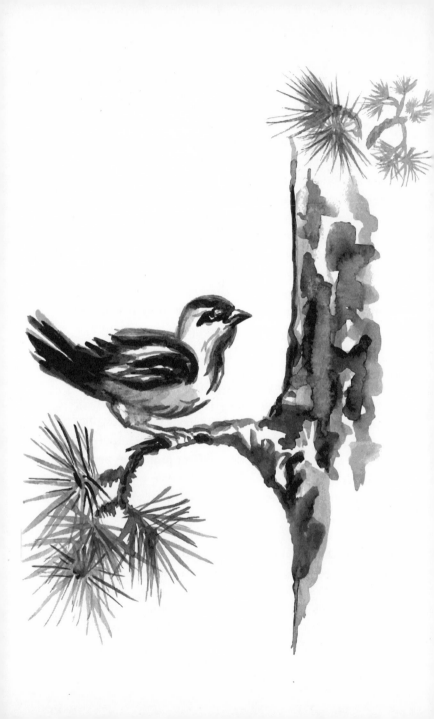

The Sounds of Nature

The popular saying "if Muhammad won't come to the mountain, then the mountain must go to Muhammad" can be applied to nature's benefits in fighting stress, anxiety and depression, even at home. In the previous chapter, we talked about plants and natural essential oils for including green therapy in our homes. What we'll be discussing in this chapter might be surprising at first, but science continues to prove the therapeutic power of birdsong. And it's not just the trill of these friendly forest dwellers that's beneficial. *BioScience* magazine echoed a study demonstrating that being able to observe birds from houses or offices helps relieve stress in those observing them.

The Therapeutic Power of Birds

The research, conducted by Daniel Cox at the University of Exeter, involved 273 volunteers from three British towns who decided to pay attention to urban birds, with surprising results. The lowest levels of anxiety and depression were measured in the respondents in the afternoon when more birds (robins, blackbirds, crows) were observed.

"This study starts to unpick the role that some key components of nature play for our mental well-being," remarked Cox, who confirmed in the study itself that people who spend less time outdoors are more vulnerable to anxious or depressive states. "Birds around the home, and nature in general, show great promise in preventative health care, making cities healthier, happier places to live," he concludes.

The Spanish Ornithological Society, SEO/BirdLife, is aware of these health advantages, and every year makes it possible for 150,000 people—children as well as adults—to participate in outdoor excursions where they observe and learn more about birds. Beyond education, groups that participate in these activities later talk about the sense of well-being and relaxation they get from these kinds of day trips. In fact, beyond observation, which promotes mindfulness and flow, the sounds of nature have been shown to quickly foster concentration and relaxation, to the point where recordings have proven to be effective with students who have trouble paying attention.

THE EXTRAORDINARY CASE OF HIKARI ŌE

Son of Nobel Prize-winner Kenzaburō Ōe, the protagonist of this amazing story was diagnosed as incompatible with life by his doctors as soon as he was born. On seeing the degree of his disability, which included serious vision and speech impairments, epilepsy, lack of physical coordination and other developmental problems, they recommended that his parents let him die.

His parents refused and, one delicate operation later, managed to keep their son alive. But the great leap in Hikari Ōe's life came one day walking in the woods with his father. He'd been attracted to birdsong early on, and his parents had given him a recording of different birds accompanied by a voice naming them. When Hikari heard a bird that day in the woods, he surprised his father by speaking for the first time, repeating the name as in the recording. This recognition of sound led his parents to hire a piano teacher for him, and he began expressing himself through delicate compositions that have since been released on records to worldwide acclaim. And it all began with the song of a bird.

Song of Serenity

A BBC article emphasized the fact that Hikari Ōe's case is not unique. There's something sublime and mysterious in birdsong that makes it highly therapeutic for human beings. While noise in the city is distracting, exhausting and makes us lose our concentration, birdsong has the opposite effect on us. Julian Treasure, chairman of The Sound Agency, asserts: "People find birdsong relaxing and reassuring because over thousands of years they have learnt when the birds sing they are safe, it's when birds stop singing that people need to worry. [...] Birdsong is also nature's alarm clock, with the dawn chorus signaling the start of the day."

This same company created a "soundtrack" with bird songs for a bank in Colombia. The bank showed a significant increase in customers opening new accounts, as well as those valuing the services they received positively, according to a survey.

The Alder Hey Children's Hospital in Liverpool has begun experimenting with sounds from nature to improve the mood of some patients. Another experiment was conducted in a primary school, also in Liverpool, in which bird songs were played after lunch when students tend to be most tired and distracted, and the children's attention spans were quickly restored. Russell Jones, one of the developers of the experiment, explained the success of the recording: "It doesn't get stuck in your head and annoy you but it doesn't lull you to sleep and bore you either. [...] I'm not sure there is any other sound that can do what birdsong does. It should be part of the soundtrack to everyone's day."

According to the experts, these natural sounds relax us while stimulating our senses because they're not repetitive. Especially when it comes to a chorus of different birds, there are no set rhythms or patterns. This tactic has even been used at Schiphol Airport in Amsterdam where a room has been created for travelers to relax before their flight with recordings of birds coming from loudspeakers hidden in real trees.

The BBC study also had a final mention for the experience of playing recorded birdsong in the restrooms of BP gas stations in Cambridgeshire to get the customers, who had complained about them, to associate them with freshness. The satisfaction level increased by 50%.

Garden of Eden at Home

All these experiences are applicable to a home environment. Long ago, many homes had canaries in cages, a cruel and unjust situation for the animals. With today's technology, there's no need to keep any songbird prisoner. We have thousands of recordings of wild birds at our disposal on YouTube and Spotify, and we can buy them from iTunes or other sites.

We can bring this natural forest "de-stressor" into our office if we need to study or balance the books, or into the living room while we enjoy reading a good book. It can be the soundtrack to our in-home yoga or meditation session, or can even lull us to sleep at nap time. Of course, nothing compares to a "live concert" of birds in their natural habitat, but just as we do with recording artists we like, a good listening session at home can calm us down and elevate our mood.

A Leaf from the Forest in Your Cup

We started this book with the story of how our adventure began, and now it's just a few pages away from ending. In this chapter, we'd like to take up a more personal thread again and relate how this four-handed effort was written with one author in Tokyo and the other in Barcelona. Besides working separately, reading scientific studies, articles and essays, and taking walks in forests to find inspiration for shinrin-yoku, we Skyped every day while we were writing, despite the eight-hour time difference, and with the same help on either side of the world: a cup of tea.

Every day at 8:15 am in Barcelona and at 4:15 pm in Tokyo, we brought to the computer table a cup of fragrant green Japanese tea. While we commented on our discoveries and discussed what to include and what to leave out of the chapter we were working on, this bittersweet herbal tea comforted and united us from 6,500 miles away. There's a whole world of feeling in a steaming bowl of tea, even if they're only leaves from the forest to warm the soul.

The Legend of Tea

Buddhism has an old story that tells of Siddhartha sitting under the bodhi tree. When he became aware of all the suffering people must face, a tear fell from his eye, and there sprouted the first tea shrub, a source of consolation in the midst of our tribulations.

However, the legendary origin of this infusion in China dates to two thousand years before Buddha. The story goes that Emperor Shen Nung discovered the benefits of tea in 2737 BCE, no less. Apparently, the emperor was asleep under a shrub while a bowl of drinking water was being boiled nearby. A little gust of wind blew some leaves from the shrub into the bowl and gave rise to the birth of the first cup of tea in history. When he brought the infusion to his lips, he was pleased by the flavor, and he soon felt himself coming out of his lethargy with renewed vigor. He immediately gave orders to his gardeners for them to identify the shrub and plant many more so that those fragrant green leaves could be enjoyed in a daily tea.

A *WABI-SABI* TEA CUP

"The most valued bowls for tea ceremony are irregularly shaped, and some have gold patches here and there, accentuating (rather than concealing) damage suffered at the hands of long-ago owners. Asymmetry and irregularity allow the possibility of growth, but perfection chokes the imagination."

Donald Keene, professor of Japanese Literature at Columbia University for more than fifty years.

The Wisdom of *Chanoyu*

Beyond whatever truth there may be to the legends, there's no doubt that tea leaves in our cup are a small expression of shinrin-yoku. And this isn't due exclusively to the well-known antioxidant power of tea, which contributes to longevity in countries where a lot of green tea is consumed. In its development over the centuries, the tea ceremony has evolved towards the simplicity and austerity that emanates from *wabi-sabi*. The ostentatious parlors of the past gave way to rustic huts with mud walls and straw roofs that were found in the middle of a garden and formed part of the ceremony because guests passed through it before going in to have tea.

This ritual, even if it's done informally with a friend or by oneself, is an invitation to be peaceful and in the present. In Japan, when tea bowls land on the table, time stops. Whoever takes part in *chanoyu*, as the tea ceremony is called in Japanese, sets aside daily worries and realizes how unique and incomparable the moment is. This is why friends who share in the tea ceremony strive to create a calm, relaxed atmosphere, which means obeying a tenet or two in the art of conversation:

- During chanoyu, any topic that might be controversial, disagreeable or stressful is to be avoided. Any matter that creates separation is excluded from tea ceremony conversation. Therefore, no one discusses politics, sports rivalries or the world's problems.
- Topics of conversation that unite the guests are encouraged instead. These could be comments on the quality and freshness of the tea and the beauty of the utensils; on the natural setting where chanoyu is taking place. Artistic discoveries may be shared, such as a good book, an exciting film, a exhibition that's not to be missed. In short, anything that can add beauty and harmony to the lives of the guests.

There are four key words that define the values governing the tea ceremony: *wa* (harmony), *kei* (respect), *sei* (purity) and *jaku* (serenity). As Kakuzo Okakura wrote in his classic *The Book of Tea*, published in the United States in 1906, "[Tea] is hygiene, for it enforces cleanliness; it is economics, for it shows comfort in simplicity rather than in the complex and costly [...] making all its votaries aristocrats in taste."

HAVE A CUP OF TEA!

Joshu, the Zen master, asked a new monk in the monastery, "Have I seen you before?"

The new monk replied, "No sir."

Joshu said, "Then have a cup of tea."

Joshu then turned to another monk, "Have I seen you here before?"

The second monk said, "Yes sir, of course you have."

Joshu said, "Then have a cup of tea."

Later the managing monk of the monastery asked Joshu, "How is it you make the same offer of tea to any reply?"

At this Joshu shouted, "Manager, are you still here?"

The manager replied, "Of course, Master."

Joshu said, "Then have a cup of tea."

—Osho, Art of Tea

Attention and Compassion

Master Joshu's repeated response may seem absurd, but it points out a feature of tea that makes it highly appreciated by Zen monks and people who meditate in general: the ability to keep us alert but not nervous, and in the present. Bear in mind that people who have trouble falling asleep shouldn't drink tea after five in the afternoon.

Paying attention doesn't just allow us to concentrate and be aware of what's going on around us. It also helps us be more present in our interactions with others. It makes us more compassionate in the Buddhist sense of the word, which doesn't mean feeling sorry for others, but acquiring enough empathy to put ourselves in someone else's place.

So an attentive, compassionate person is fully in the moment while listening, which is the greatest gift we can offer someone who opens their heart to us. The kind of intense listening that tea drinking encourages also happens on one's own. Many great ideas and decisions have been made alone, thanks to the focus bestowed by a cup of tea.

Incidentally, thank you for your attention, and for accompanying us all this way. Once we've gone over some of the principles discussed in these pages, it will be time to close the book and open the door to nature, where the pulse of life waits.

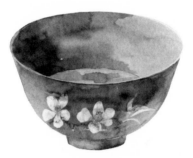

EPILOGUE

The 10 Principles of *Shinrin-yoku* for Everyday Living

We'll get the most out of these pages by ending our journey with ten principles.

ONE ━━━ Bathe in Greenery Once a Week

Science has shown that the health benefits of shinrin-yoku last for several days until we next submerge ourselves in the forest.

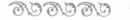

TWO ━━━ Live Mindfully

The serenity and wealth of stimulation found in nature make it an excellent training ground for mindfulness and for opening our perception up to all five senses.

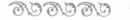

THREE ━━━ Hug a Tree

There's a belief going back to the ancient Celts that being in contact with a living tree recharges us while at the same time easing our tensions and anxieties.

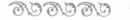

FOUR ━━━ "Listen to the Birds Sing"

Numerous studies have shown that birdsong, even when recorded, is therapeutic and enhances concentration, confidence and relaxation.

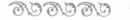

FIVE ━━━ Walk with No Direction in Mind

Once you pass nature's gates, forget about being rushed. Like any good traveler, don't try to get anywhere in particular; let your feet and your inspiration lead you.

SIX ━━━ Stop and Breathe
Science has proven that the phytoncides given off by nature increase our defenses against numerous diseases, as well as lifting our spirits.

SEVEN ━━━ Write a Haiku
We can take home a bit of the forest by capturing the moment in a short, hand-written poem, or we can immortalize what we see by sketching it in a notebook.

EIGHT ━━━ Let *Wabi-sabi* Inspire You
In nature, nothing is perfect, nothing is finished, nothing is forever. "The beauty of imperfections" teaches us to accept ourselves and to see our failings as an opportunity for growth.

NINE ━━━ Have a Cup of Tea
After a pleasant walk in nature, but also during a break in our working day, a brew made with leaves from the forest will restore our vitality as well as encouraging mindfulness.

TEN ━━━ Feel the *Yugen*
Experience the pleasure and deep connection of being one with nature through meditation, whether sitting, lying down or being aware of each step you take. You are part of the universe and the universe is you.

BIBLIOGRAPHY

Other Books by the Same Authors
Miralles, Francesc, and Héctor García. *Ikigai: the Japanese Secret to a Long and Happy Life*. New York, Penguin Books 2017 [Original edition: *Ikigai: los secretos de Japón para una vida larga y feliz*. Madrid: Urano, 2016.]
— *The Ikigai Journey: a Practical Guide to Finding Happiness and Purpose the Japanese Way*. North Clarendon, Vermont: Tuttle Publishing, 2020. [Original edition: *El método Ikigai: despierta tu verdadera pasión y cumple tus propósitos vitals*. Barcelona: Aguilar, 2017.]

Miralles, Francesc. *Wabi-sabi*. Barcelona. B de Bolsillo (Ediciones B), 2014.

García, Héctor. *A Geek in Japan: Discovering the Land of Manga, Anime, Zen and the Tea Ceremony*. North Clarendon, Vermont: Tuttle Publishing, 2011, 2019 [Original edition: *Un Geek en Japón*. Barcelona: Norma Editorial, 2012.]

Texts by Other Authors
Bachelard, Gaston. *La poética del espacio, Fondo de Cultura Económica*. México D. F., 2010.

Cali, Joseph, and John Dougill. *Shinto Shrines: A Guide to the Sacred Sites of Japan's Ancient Religion*. Honolulu: Latitude 20 (University of Hawaii Press), 2012.

Gardiner, Joey. "City-dwellers are prone to depression—are high-rises to blame?"

The Guardian, March 16, 2017.

Gold, Taro. *Living Wabi Sabi: The True Beauty of Your Life*. Kansas City: Andrews McMeel, 2004.

Hesse, Hermann. *El caminante*. Barcelona: Bruguera, 1986.

Juniper, Andrew. *Wabi Sabi: The Japanese Art of Imperma-nence*. North Clarendon, Vermont: Tuttle Publishing, 2003.

Kabat-Zinn, Jon. *Vivir con plenitud las crisis: cómo utilizar la sabiduría del cuerpo y de la mente para enfrentarnos al estrés, el dolor y la enfermedad*. Barcelona: Kairós, 2016.

Koren, Leonard. *Wabi-sabi para artistas, diseñadores, poetas y filósofos*, Barcelona: Sd, 2015.

Martín Asuero, Andrés. *Con rumbo propio: disfruta de la vida sin estrés*. Barcelona: Plataforma, 2010.

Milner, Marion. *A Life of One's Own*. New York: Routledge, 2011.

Muir, John. *The Yosemite*. WLC Books, 2009.
—*My First Summer in the Sierra*. St. Louis, Missouri : J. Missouri, 2013.
—*The Mountains of California*. Wanderlust, 2015.

Nhat Hanh, Thich. *El milagro del mindfulness*. Barcelona: Oniro, 2013.

Okakura, Kakuzo. *El libro del té*. (Okakura).

Osho. *El arte del té: meditaciones para despertar tu espíritu*. Móstoles: Gaia, 2007.

Quan, Diana. *El paraíso es tu casa*. Barcelona: B de Books (Ediciones B), 2017.

Silverstone, Matthew. *Blinded by Science*. London. Lloyd's World Publishing, 2011.

Sompayrac, Lauren M. *How the inmune system works*. Hoboken: Wiley-Blackwell, 2015.

Taleb, Nassim Nicholas. *Antifrágil: las cosas que se benefician del desorden*. Barcelona: Paidós, 2013.

Tanizaki, Junichiro. *El elogio de la sombra*. Madrid: Siruela, 2010.

Thoreau, Henry David.*Walden and Civil Disobedience*. New York: Penguin Books, 2017 ed.
—*Walking*. New York: Cosmo, Inc, 2006 ed.

Tokyo Metabolism 2010: 50 Years After 1960. Encyclopedia vol. I.

Scientific Articles by Theme
General Science on *Shurin-yoku*

Hansen, Margaret M., Reo Jones, and Kirsten Tocchini. "*Shinrin-yoku* (Forest Bathing) and Nature Therapy: A State-of-the-Art Review." International Journal of Environmental Research and Public Health 14, no. 8 (July 28, 2017): 851. https://doi.org/10.3390/ijerph14080851.

Lee, Juyoung, Qing Li, Liisa Tyrvinen, Yuko Tsunetsugu, Bum-Jin Park, Takahide Kagawa, and Yoshifumi Miyazaki. "Nature Therapy and Preventive Medicine." In Public Health - Social and Behavioral Health, published by Jay Maddock. InTech, 2012. https://doi.org/10.5772/37701.

Science of Phytoncides

Park, Bum-Jin, Yuko Tsunetsugu, Tamami Kasetani, Takahide Kagawa, and Yoshifumi Miyazaki. "The Physiological Effects of *Shinrin-yoku* (Taking in the Forest Atmosphere or Forest Bathing): Evidence from Field Experiments in 24 Forests across Japan." Environmental Health and Preventive Medicine 15, no. 1 (January, 2010): 18-26. https://doi.org/10.1007/s12199-009-0086-9.

Park, Bum-Jin, Yuko Tsunetsugu, Tamami Kasetani, Hideki Hirano, Takahide Kagawa, Masahiko Sato, and Yoshifumi Miyazaki. "Physiological Effects of *Shinrin-yoku* (Taking in the Atmosphere of the Forest) — Using Salivary Cortisol and Cerebral Activity as Indicators —." Journal of Physiological Anthropology 26, no. 2 (2007): 123-28. https://doi.org/10.2114/jpa2.26.123.

Science of Houseplants

Lee, Min-sun, Juyoung Lee, Bum-Jin Park, and Yoshifumi Miyazaki. "Interaction with Indoor Plants May Reduce Psychological and Physiological Stress by Suppressing Autonomic Nervous System Activity in Young Adults: A Randomized Crossover Study." Journal of Physiological Anthropology 34, no. 1 (December, 2015). https://doi.org/10.1186/s40101-015-0060-8.

Wolverton, B. C., Douglas, Willard L., and Keith Bounds. "Clean Air Study. A study of interior landscape plants for indoor air pollution abatement." NASA, 1989.

Science of Aromatherapy

Dayawansa, Samantha, Katsumi Umeno, Hiromasa Takakura, Etsuro Hori, Eiichi Tabuchi, Yoshinao Nagashima, Hiroyuki Oosu, et al. "Autonomic Responses during Inhalation of Natural Fragrance of "Cedrol" in Humans." Autonomic Neuroscience 108, no. 1-2 (October, 2003): 79-86. https://doi.org/10.1016/j.autneu.2003.08.002.

ACKNOWLEDGEMENTS

OUR THANKS

TO SANDRA AND BERTA BRUNA, who to date have sown the seed of our *Ikigai* in 40 of the world's languages.

TO ALL OF OUR PUBLISHERS, for transmitting the wisdom of Japan to the four corners of the world.

TO ORIOL ALCORTA, Spanish publisher of this book, for having placed his trust in us and in this beautiful project.

TO JUN MATSUURA, illustrator of the Spanish edition, who has drunk from the pure fountains of *sumi-e*.

TO VICTOR JURADO, our head historian.

TO OUR FAMILIES and friends.

TO VICENTE, ROSA, AITOR, RODRIGO AND CARLOS, for their corrections and support at all times.

TO EVERYONE WHO READ *Ikigai* and *The Ikigai Journey*, for making this new book possible.

PHOTO CREDITS

All illustrations/photographs in this book are from Shutterstock.com on the pages listed below:-